Notes on Paediatric Dentistry

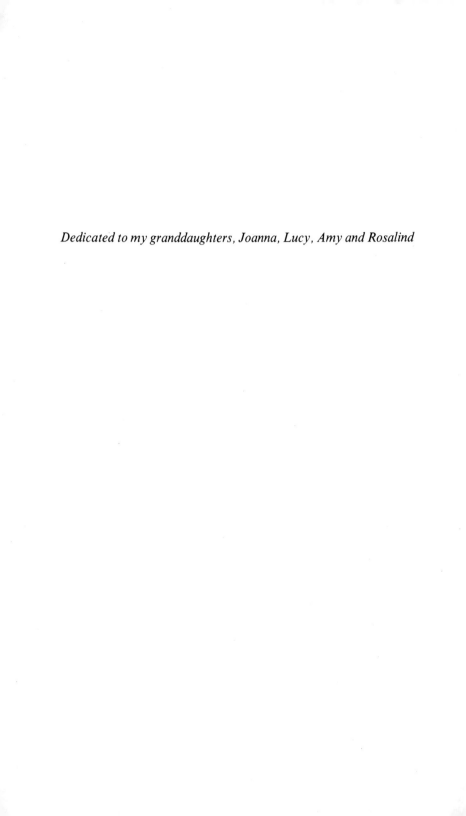

Dedicated to my granddaughters, Joanna, Lucy, Amy and Rosalind

Notes on Paediatric Dentistry

Stanley F. Parkin, MDS(Lond.), FDS, RCS(Eng.)
Senior Lecturer and Honorary Consultant in Children's Dentistry,
Head of the Children's Dentistry Department, Vice Dean and
Clinical Tutor, University College and Middlesex School of
Dentistry, London

Wright

Wright
An imprint of Butterworth–Heinemann Ltd
Halley Court, Jordan Hill, Oxford OX2 8EJ

Oxford London Guildford Boston Munich New Delhi Singapore Sydney
Tokyo Toronto Wellington

 PART OF REED INTERNATIONAL P.L.C.

First published 1991

British Library Cataloguing in Publication Data
Parkin, S. F. (Stanley Frederick)
Notes on paediatric dentistry.
1. Dentistry
I. Title
617.645

ISBN 0-7236-1643-4

Library of Congress Cataloging in Publication Data
Parkin, S. F.
Notes on paediatric dentistry/Stanley F. Parkin.
p.   cm.
Includes bibliographical references
Includes index.
ISBN 0-7236-1643-4 : $13.95
1. Pedodontics. I. Title.
[DNLM: 1. Pedodontics. WU 480 P247n]
RK55.C5P37 1991
617.6′45—dc20
DNLM/DLC
for Library of Congress

Photoset by BC Typesetting, Bristol BS15 5YS
Printed in Great Britain by BPCC Wheatons Ltd, Exeter

Preface

This short book aims to bring together the main core subject matter of Paedodontics, or Children's Dentistry. It is intended to be of use to both the undergraduate student preparing for the Final examination and the busy practitioner seeking a rapid 'update'. Editorial policy has been to keep the references to a minimum, but indications are given for further reading.

As the author, I am acutely aware of several things. The first is that, as John Miller wrote, in the present academic climate it is extremely difficult to get experts to agree about the details of their specialty. Accordingly, I have attempted to seek and report the 'middle ground' and if possible to avoid the controversial and obscure.

Secondly, I need to acknowledge the enormous debt I owe to all the sources of knowledge and learning and experience that have been available to me over the years: teachers, libraries, journals, contemporaries, hospital and nursing staff, students, dental surgery assistants, parents and not least the children themselves.

Finally, I must record my gratitude to Dr Geoffrey Smaldon and Mrs Lucy Sayer of Butterworth Scientific for their support, encouragement and practical advice during the writing of this book, to many friends and colleagues who have read and commented on the manuscript, and to my wife and family without whom I would never have found the time and endurance to complete it.

Footnotes
1. The word 'paedodontics' is derived from the Greek *paes*—the child, and *odus*—the tooth.
2. Throughout the book I have referred to the child as 'he' in order to avoid the clumsy 'he/she' option.

Contents

Chapter 1

The child

Introduction

A general understanding of children, childhood, child psychology and the philosophies of child care is essential for the successful practice of paedodontics. Dental care cannot be carried out in isolation from the rest of an individual child's existence and experience without the risk of unwittingly creating unnecessary problems, stresses and difficulties for all concerned.

The aims of child care

The proper aim of everyone responsible for the care of a child is to promote its best physical and mental health, while remaining constantly alert to recognize, prevent, cure or mitigate any condition that might mar or handicap the full potential growth and development of the child's body, mind or personality.

The essential needs of childhood

Mary Sheridan (1975) outlined concisely the fundamental needs of a growing child: 'All children, normal and abnormal, progressing from the helplessness of infancy to the independence of maturity, have certain physical needs, without which life itself cannot continue, and certain psychological needs, without which an individual cannot obtain contentment, self-reliance and good relationships with other people.

'Basic physical needs
There can be little disagreement about these seven essentials for existence:
   shelter and protective care;
   food;
   warmth and clothing;

fresh air and sunlight;
activity and rest;
prevention of illness or injury;
training in habits and skills necessary for the maintenance of
    life.'   .

'Basic psychological needs

These relate to both intellectual and emotional development because
they are so closely interwoven that it is difficult to provide for them
adequately except in combination. They include:
affection and continuity of individual care;
security rooted in a knowledge of belonging, in stable personal
    relationships and in familiar environmental surroundings;
a sense of personal identity, dignity as a human being, and
    self-respect derived from knowledge of being valued as an
    individual;
opportunity to learn from experience;
opportunity to achieve success in some field of endeavour
    however small;
opportunity to achieve independence, personal and so far as
    possible, financial;
opportunity to take responsibility and be of service to others.'

Monitoring progress

To study, monitor and care for a child the areas of physical, mental,
emotional and social growth and development are taken into
account.

Numerous growth tables, charts and nomograms (e.g. Buckler,
1979; Tanner and Whitehouse, 1983, and Inslay, 1986) have been
published in an attempt to provide standard milestones that the
child may be expected to reach at certain ages.

Paediatric growth charts plot the average physical growth in
height and weight percentiles against age. They also give indications
of growth velocities at each age. In general there are two growth
spurts. First there is a rapid but decelerating increase in height and
weight from birth to 2 years. This is followed by a steady but
gradually slowing velocity until at puberty there is another acceler-
ation of height growth (in girls aged 12–13½ years, and boys aged
13–15½ years) which ceases at sexual maturity when the long bone
epiphyses fuse. The limbs grow faster than the trunk and this
changes the body proportions of the older child.

Body weight and height have similar growth rates in each individual, but will be affected by health, nutrition, genetics and

environmental factors. (A rough guide to adult height is that it will be twice that of child at age 2 years ± 2 cm (Illingworth, 1983)).

Failure to reach these norms or averages may be a developmental warning sign. However, some caution has to be maintained about interpreting such targets too literally. Illingworth (1983) said that in the assessment of an individual child whose measurements are unusual, its size at birth and the build of its parents are the chief non-disease factors to be considered. Of far greater importance than the child's height and weight are its well-being, abundant energy, happiness, freedom from infection and freedom from lassitude. If these are apparent then the child is unlikely to have serious organic disease. Thus when considering any aspect of a child's physical growth it is important to learn about parents, hereditary factors, intra-uterine environment, problems at birth, and feeding and health in infancy.

There are also many graded tests for visual and auditory acuity, disorders of communication, and of personality or social adjustment.

Developmental assessment scales have been produced by Gesell (1938, 1947), Sheridan (1975) and Illingworth (1983).

Sheridan based her valuable assessment tool for children up to the age of five years on the consideration of the four outstanding human achievements: upright locomotion, hand–eye coordination, use of spoken language and the evolution of a complex social culture. By listing in detail many of the expected levels of activity and ability at each age it provides a sensible baseline with which to compare an individual child. The items in themselves are simple statements, e.g. 'Age 6 months: Hearing and Speech: Turns immediately to mother's voice across the room.' Together they form a comprehensive battery. A child does not Pass or Fail in this respect, but the assessor would be concerned if it did not respond positively to approximately two-thirds of the items listed in each of the four sections.

It is important that every child is closely monitored at every stage from birth onwards. This is normally done within the family and in close partnership with the health professionals, health visitors, child health clinics and social workers. Usually pre-school children are screened from time to time by the general health service and later by the school medical service. (These health agencies also give and offer advice and support, arrange care in the event of accident or illness, and initiate routine immunization against communicable diseases.) Unmistakable motor disability, mental retardation or psychological or social problems demand immediate referral for specialized opinion and care.

Early screening and careful management mean that 'damaged'

children are surviving longer to maturity and doctors and dentists are becoming more experienced and better equipped to deal with such children's special problems.

Psychological theory

Psychology is the science of behaviour and mental processes. (Psychiatry is concerned with mental health and illness.) Beginning with the ancient philosophers psychology has evolved, often influenced by contemporary thought and discoveries, to examine and theorize about human and animal nature and the visible and invisible workings of the mind. However, it is only relatively recently that the demands of scientific proof and replication of results have begun to grow and thus many areas of modern psychological theory are still empiric.

Modern schools of psychology approach the subject from a variety of diverse viewpoints (Atkinson *et al.*, 1990):

1. Neurobiological. Linking behaviour and mental events to the processes of neurobiology.
2. Behavioural. Supports the theory of Stimulus–Response (S–R) and Operant Conditioning (see later). Behavioural studies tend towards recorded observation, tests and scales and the process of obtaining numerical values that allow statistical evaluation.
3. Cognitive. Concerned with perception, imagery, problem solving, remembering, information processing.
4. Psychoanalytical. The effects on behaviour of unconscious beliefs, fears and desires. Investigation involves talking to the individual and using the trained practitioner to interpret what he says.
5. Phenomenological. Concerned with subjective feelings, training and teaching children. Studies how people view themselves: self-concept, self-esteem, self-awareness and humanistic mental qualities that distinguish man from animals.

Although all of these schools may throw some light upon a child's reactions in the dental situation, the most helpful theories of explanation so far have been influenced strongly by the Psychoanalytical and Behavioural views, both of which agree that human personality is greatly influenced for good or ill by experiences during childhood or infancy.

Freud (1856–1939), the pioneer of psychoanalysis, visualized the human personality as an iceberg with only its tip, the conscious experience, above the surface while the unconscious, filled with primitive passions and impulses, still exerted a large influence on the subject's reactions.

He postulated a theory of personality development with a tripartite unconscious personality composed of:

The *id*: the unconscious deep-seated instinct and impulses and social and aggressive drives not under the control of reason.

The *ego*: that part of the personality which assesses reality through the five senses and assesses the bodily environment and directs behaviour accordingly.

The *super-ego*: the conscience, which provides the moral judgements and opposition to the id.

He suggested that between birth and the age of 3 years many basic strivings, emotional conflicts and motives have their beginnings. In his opinion, during this period, libidinous energy is focused on various body zones: Age $0-1\frac{1}{2}$ years: oral; Age $1\frac{1}{2}-3$ years: anal; Age 3–6 years: genital.

Thus Freudians view the mouth as a human organ of desire, pleasure and satisfaction for the infant citing the close association between hunger, breast sucking, food and contentment. In later years the mouth remains a centre of emotional expression and satisfaction: kissing, smoking, eating, drinking, aggression, speaking and spitting.

The trained Freudian analyst seeks to interpret and understand the subject's basic elements of personality by exploring the unconscious using free association (talking of everything that comes into the conscious mind), the discussion of childhood experiences and dream recall.

Watson, in the early 20th century, introduced the ideas of Behaviourism which sought observable and measurable data from psychological studies in order to achieve a more scientific basis of research. Thus he and his followers (including Skinner, b. 1904) attacked the introspective approach of the Psychoanalysts and concentrated on what the subject actually did. Stimulus–Response psychology takes note of the effects of the rewards and punishments that elicit specific responses from the subject under observation and also how behaviour may be modified by changing the patterns of stimulation.

Classical conditioning occurs when a subject learns that one event is always followed by another, e.g. for a baby the sight of the breast is followed by the taste of milk.

Operant conditioning is where, for example, a rat in a Skinner box learns to operate a bar which releases a pellet of food and the arrival of the food reinforces the bar pressing. The specific desired response is immediately rewarded. If the bar-pressing stops delivering the desired pellet, the reflex response is gradually extinguished.

From an understanding of these simple basic ideas it is possible to begin to appreciate complex studies of behaviour shaping, reinforcement of appropriate behaviour, and secondary reinforcement by a 'daisy chain' of linked events.

Piaget (1932 *et seq.*) focused on the cognitive intellectual development of the child as follows:

1. Sensorimotor: 0–2 years
   Becomes aware of the relationship between his actions and the effect on the environment.
2. Pre-operational: 2–7 years
   Uses language, images, words, and is egocentric.
3. Concrete operational: 7–12 years
   Becomes capable of logical thought. Begins to recognize relational terms (e.g. A < B), numbers, sizes, weights, classifications.
4. Formal operational: 12+ years
   Can think in abstract and reason systematically. Becomes concerned with hypothetical concepts and the future.

Erikson (1963) described the child passing through a series of psychosocial stages that represent a widening of human relationships (mother:parents:family:school:peer groups) as its personality developed.

Anxiety and fear

The behavioural effects of anxiety and fear can become serious barriers to the delivery of dental care because they lead to non-attendance, failed appointments, and poor cooperation and disruptive behaviour in the dental chair. A basic understanding of these normal emotions can help the dental surgeon and his staff to prevent, minimize or overcome their effect on children in the dental surgery.

Definitions

Anxiety
A painful uneasiness of mind over an impending or anticipated ill, often coupled with a feeling of tightness and distress in the precordial region; to press, to strangle. Freud (1922) wrote that 'anxiety itself needs no description; everyone has experienced this sensation, or to speak more correctly this affective condition, at

some time or other'. Anxiety may be described as 'fear spread thin'. Spielberger (1966) differentiated between A-Trait and A-State anxiety, for anxiety may be considered to be free-floating or specific. To a great extent Dental Anxiety falls into the second category for it arises most acutely at a particular moment in association with a particular event or environment.

Fear
A normal response in higher animals to an active or imagined threat plus unpleasant subjective feelings of terror. The physiological response is that of 'fight or flight'. It is particularly acute when the subject is helpless.

Phobia
A special kind of fear that is out of proportion to the situation, which cannot be explained or reasoned away, is beyond voluntary control, and which leads to an avoidance of the feared situation, e.g. the dental surgery. (*Phobos:* A Greek god who could strike fear into one's enemies.)

Aetiology

Basic fears
Certain inbuilt fears and anxieties are thought to arise from a very primal period of evolution, serving to maintain the individual's life and integrity by causing him to avoid potentially damaging things and circumstances and to react rapidly in the face of threat. It has been suggested there are several easily understood and quite normal fears and anxieties in modern subjects of all ages, which although they have useful protective effects, are more appropriate and suitable for the tree-top jungle existence (Marks, 1969). Unfortunately many of them can be cued in the dental chair.

1. Fear of the unknown. This is manifested in a special care and defence in the presence of strange and unexplored environments, strange persons or objects, and in fear of the dark. These fears are particularly intense if the subject is lost or alone. A baby forms a strong security attachment to its mother or mother-substitute and, until about 3 years old, becomes distressed if separated from them in a strange situation (separation anxiety).
2. Fear of heights. The subject must be protected from the possibility of falling. In common with many small animals, even from an early age a child will be afraid of being in such a

situation or near a 'visual step' perceived as the edge of a precipice.

3. Fear of loss of support. The unexpected unpleasant sensation of falling is frightening. Yet perversely some children like the excitement of being swung about by someone that they trust and who cares for them, and they will giggle with delight. (This is a good example of how some individuals, by overcoming a basic fear and experiencing it again and again without actually suffering any harm, begin to enjoy and seek the stimulation, e.g. in parachuting, fairground rides, etc.)

4. Fear of being stared at. This action, resembling the intensity of an animal staring at its potential prey before attacking it, may make a child feel ill at ease and even fearful.

5. Fear of the 'hawk effect' of something hovering over one's head. Again this cues the fear of attack.

6. Fear of the exposure of the ventral surface of the body (such as when a patient lies supine in the dental chair). This is fear-provoking because it leaves the soft underbelly exposed and vulnerable. For many animals this is a signal of total surrender and submission ('Hands Up!').

7. Fear of the invasion of personal space by having a stranger in extremely close proximity. This intimacy can only be allowed to persons who are particularly privileged and trustworthy, e.g. family, loved ones, hairdresser, doctor, dentist (Argyle, 1975). Not every child has learned the fine distinction that it is safe and correct to allow the professional as close to them as this.

8. Fear of bodily mutilation or pain. While small children are strongly affected by separation anxiety, older children are generally more concerned about the danger of injury, sharp objects, bleeding and pain. From puberty boys are said to suffer from a form of castration anxiety in the dental chair for fear of losing valuable masculine teeth.

Learned fears

Fears may also be learned from experiences, real or imagined, first and secondhand, and social fears can be enhanced if they are used by parents to train the child to behave appropriately. ('Don't do that, everyone is staring at you!' or 'Brush your teeth or the dentist will want to pull them all out!').

These very short paragraphs of exploration are included to give the new reader a little of the flavour of this fascinating subject of psychology in the hope that they will be stimulated and encouraged to read more widely, e.g. for a general introduction, Atkinson *et al*. (1990).

Stages of childhood development

The following tables include a few items that are of direct value to the dental surgeon. They are not, of course, to be regarded as a screening system.

Age 0-1   Baby

Physical
In developed countries such as the UK the average baby boy weighs, at birth, 7 lb 4 oz (2.9 kg) and the average girl slightly less. A baby born 4–5 weeks before the normal 280 days (10 lunar months) of pregnancy have elapsed is classified as premature. Any baby weighing under 5 lb 8 oz (2.2 kg) is considered to be a low birth weight baby and needs intensive care. One child in 48 is born with a congenital deformity. The first month of a child's life is one of the most critical for survival.

The newborn is helpless and very dependent on mother and on the regular appearance of food and mother love. It clings on to its mother with hands and feet and matches her pulse rate if she is frightened.

The baby's physical development may be affected by antenatal influences.

Motor activity
Feeding takes priority. The first oral experiences may have future psychological significance for dental care.

Feeding the baby
Breast feeding. This method has several advantages. It is cheap, 'producer to consumer', with reduced chances of gastroenteritis and respiratory infections. It increases bonding between the mother and baby and gives the child contentment, security and protection. This contentment leads to non-nutritive sucking and perhaps predisposes to thumb-sucking or the use of a pacifier (dummy) in later months.

The composition of breast milk varies from day to day and feed to feed. The mother's state of nutrition affects the quality. Drugs which the mother is taking can be passed to the baby in the milk, e.g. alcohol, tobacco, barbiturates, indomethicin, tetracycline, anticoagulants. Weaning from breast to bottle or cup and spoon is usually not later than 6–7 months. Breast feeding is sometimes continued longer when, from an old wives' tale, the mother expects that the delayed ovulation associated with milk production may have a contraceptive effect. This is not always the case, however. Parents must be made aware that in some cases, breast feeding on demand can be a causative factor in dental caries as the child's teeth erupt.

Artificial feeding. Problems can arise when the mother is unable or unwilling to breast feed, and bottle feeding is substituted. Breast feeding is a basic instinct but bottle feeding gives the mother more freedom.

Bottle feeding breaks the mother–mouth–comfort–protection links and other people can now feed the baby. The feed has to be carefully prepared and sterilized. Delays can occur at normal feeding times thus keeping the hungry child frustrated and unhappy. Cow's milk differs considerably in composition from human milk and cow's milk products in baby foods are 'humanized'. They must be diluted properly for overconcentrated feeds of condensed or powdered milk can cause fits and brain damage. There is a danger of underfeeding or overfeeding and infected feeding bottles or teats can cause gastroenteritis.

The baby starts to take soft, puréed food at about 4 months and begins to chew at about 7 months.

Ideally the child should be weaned to drinking from a cup by the age of 1 year, but unfortunately some parents continue to give the older infant a bottle for comfort reasons and to get it off to sleep. If the bottle now contains anything other than plain water the erupted teeth will decay rapidly (bottle caries), commencing with the upper incisors and proceeding to the posterior teeth. The lower incisors are often the last to be affected.

Sensory activity

Hearing and sight are developing. By the 4th month the baby is attempting vocalization to gain attention. If undetected deafness is present the child gives up these vocal attempts by the 8th month and may suffer speech problems in the future.

Communication

By crying for attention.

Social

There is a change in family outlook for the baby requires considerable expenditure of time and effort from the parents in 24 hour attention and care.

Dental/oral
The baby should be examined to ensure early detection and care of any abnormalities, e.g. cleft palate. Systemic disturbances can cause permanent irregularities in the calcification of the teeth. Decisions should be taken during the first year about the need to give fluoride supplements. Psychologists are aware of the significance of the mouth in the development of the emotions with regard to feeding, comfort and contentment.

Age 1   Infant

Physical
Weight since birth triples. Still needs nappies day and night. Teeth erupting.

Motor activity
Drinks from a cup. Sits up without support. Crawls. Attempts to stand and can stand supported by furniture. Can walk with feet wide apart with someone holding its hand.
Age 15 months: Can feed itself.

Sensory activity
Localizes sounds and responds to its name. Eyes follow moving objects; recognizes familiar people.

Communication
Afraid of strange surroundings and people, clings to mother. Points at things and explores items by biting or chewing them.
Age 15–18 months: Speaks jargon, perhaps five words, but understands more.

Social
Understands simple commands, shakes head for 'no', waves 'bye bye'. Affectionate.

Dental/oral
Suffers the problems of painful teething. Commence care of the erupting teeth. Stop bottle feeding. The mother should be given additional advice about avoiding a caries-promoting diet for her child and shown how to clean its teeth. There is an increasing incidence of traumatic injuries to the teeth in this age group as children fall while learning to walk.

Age 2–3   Toddler

Physical
Out of nappies during day.

Motor activity
Can climb up and down stairs. Jumps. Can ride a tricycle. Begins to change from whole hand palm grip to more precise finger and thumb movement. Can draw.

Sensory activity
Hearing and sight now fully developed.

Communication
Age 2 years: 300-word vocabulary. Uses three word phrases.
Age 3 years: 900-word vocabulary. Uses five word sentences. Knows own first and last name.

Social
Age 2 years: Has tantrums when frustrated. Clings to mother in affection, tiredness and fear. Depends on mother, is jealous of her attention and can suffer separation anxiety when she is not there. Fearful of strangers.

In the dental surgery: Shy at first. Needs time to adjust in new surroundings. The dentist should use simple commands and questions and follow the routine of 'Tell, Show, Do'. 'Cooperation time' must not be wasted in delays that keep child waiting.

Age 2½ years: Increasing independence. Self-assertive. 'I can do it!'. In the dental surgery: Ready to refuse to cooperate. May say 'NO!' to every suggestion. The dentist should not ask for cooperation directly, but rather give false choices. 'Which bur shall I use for your tooth?' Delaying tactics should not be allowed.

Age 3 years: More amenable. Helps. Easier to control with words ('special', 'secret', 'surprise', 'different', 'magic' and so on can be very useful). Has reasoning and initiative.

In the dental surgery: At this age particularly the child must never be left alone and unsupervised for he will probably begin to explore his surroundings and may get into trouble.

Dental/oral
Primary teeth have erupted and need preventive monitoring and

care. The child cannot brush its own teeth yet but wants to help. The mother should brush the child's teeth first and then allow him to 'finish them off'. Toothbrushing should be fun and not a battle. Reinforce diet, oral hygiene and fluoride advice.

Age 4–5   Pre-school

Physical
Height since birth doubles.

Motor activity
Walks down stairs using alternate feet.
Age 5: Eats well with knife and fork, ties own shoelaces.

Communication
By now has a 2000-word vocabulary, and uses sentences of six–eight words. Can identify and describe items. Drawings become more recognizable. Asks questions continually.

Social
Age 4 years: Active, talkative, dogmatic and boastful. Sense of personal identity developing. Appreciates 'man to man' conversation. In the dental surgery: Be firm and fair, give a lot of praise. Answer all those 'What's that for?' questions as you work and try to avoid the child's delaying tactics.
Age 5 years: Speech is fluent. Socially sensible, controlled, and independent. Likes to attend to one thing at a time, is composed, can tolerate discomfort.
Over 90% of under fives go to day nursery, nursery class of primary schools, nursery schools, play groups or child minders. Thus many of them are learning self-control, to conform, to overcome separation anxiety when away from mother, and to respond to other caring adults.

Age 6–12   School age

Physical
Active with increased manual and bodily dexterity. Pre-puberty changes begin to appear at the end of this period.

Motor activity
Age 6 years: Draws and paints well.
Age 7 years: Practises well in order to gain desired skills.
Age 8 years: Motor control well developed. Can use tools, e.g. hammer and screwdriver.

Communication
Vocabulary expands to over 2500 words. Uses complex sentences. Uses words well.

Social
Increasingly interested in hobbies, skills, sports. Makes collections of items and information. Extends experience beyond the family into the larger school group. Becomes more stoical and able to conceal feelings. Fears blood and mutilation more than separation.

Periods of self-critical doubts, especially about body image and appearance.

Dental/oral
Losing milk teeth and going through the 'ugly duckling' period. Can brush teeth well. Good period for teaching detail and science of dental care. Fissure sealing of permanent teeth and possible need for orthodontic treatment should be considered.

Age 13–18   Adolescent

Physical
Pubertal changes and hormonal changes. Undergoes a growth spurt. Becomes very aware of changing facial features and body. May feel clumsy, awkward and ungainly.

Motor activity
Refining motor skills.

Communication
Now has adult proficiency with words, but uses slang with peers.

Social
A period of special difficulties for most children.

With growing intelligence they tend to become opinionated and argumentative, and feel that they must test everything, e.g. love, strength, emotive needs, authority.

They usually have absolute confidence that they are right about everything and that their judgement is infallible. They may come into conflict with parents over parents' 'mistakes' for they are not sophisticated enough to make allowances.

They may undergo strains of important school examinations and parental ambition.

The individual feels the need to conform with his peers: gang, group, 'crazes'. He seeks independence and underlines this by rejection of old ways and values.

Tends to choose clothes that help him to get comfortable with new physical changes and appearance.

Becomes aware of the teenage problems associated with sexual development: how to acquire correct knowledge, keep up with perceived social norms, and how to cope with feelings.

Dental/oral
The adolescent should be capable of achieving good oral hygiene, have knowledge of the dietary causes of dental caries and can accept more prolonged treatment procedures. However, this can become a period of increasing caries incidence because of neglect of good oral hygiene habits and the personal choice of rapid energy, high sugar content, food and drink for sports etc. The dentist should reinforce the preventive measures, and monitor oral hygiene and dental and periodontal condition regularly. During this period the appearance becomes increasingly important to the adolescent and this can be a valuable lever for motivating dental care programmes again. Boys tend to fail dental appointments more often than girls.

Chapter 2

Behaviour management in the dental surgery

Looked at realistically, the dentist's conception of a perfect standard of child behaviour in the dental surgery is unobtainable.

From the start he wants to see a quiet, quickly-cooperative child who is willing to allow a stranger to look inside his mouth under a bright light and to use disagreeable means to examine and treat his teeth. He wants his patient to put up with a dry mouth, loud noises, unpleasant tastes and unfamiliar sensations, needles, drills and other unknown and unimaginable items while remaining at ease in unfamiliar surroundings and not causing any delays or interruptions. Finally at the end of a prolonged treatment session he wants the child to fully appreciate his efforts and to be thankful.

This asks for an impossible level of collaboration for most youngsters, and yet there are many practitioners, perhaps preoccupied with their operative techniques, who feel a profound sense of failure when they do not achieve many of these conditions when treating a child.

When first considering behavioural management in dentistry another problem must be identified. Dental surgeons, from their scientific, practical background are conditioned to seek a neat, orderly structure and sequential explanation to clinical problems with direct, definite instructions about how to overcome them. The management of children cannot be described in this way because it is a living, changing interaction of many factors. These will include the child's age, personality, past experience, parental training, imagination, misinterpretation, and so on, let alone the confrontation with the unfamiliar dental surgery treatment situation.

However, much can be done by thought, empathy, rehearsal and understanding to develop a comfortable personal style together with the ability to adapt successfully to the many subtle differences between young patients and the moment-to-moment changes that will occur during an individual child's visit to the dental practice.

Behaviour management in dental surgery can be focused on three main areas:

1. The child.
2. The dental practice.
3. The care procedure.

The child

A child's introduction to the whole subject of dental care begins at home where the family's attitudes to diet, care of the teeth and dental treatment are quickly learned and accepted as the norm. The child's life style, general experiences both vicarious and first-hand, and the way in which it is taught and helped to come to terms with inevitable life experiences will obviously affect his reactions in the dental surgery. (Thus the 'conditioning' of the child is the responsibility of the parent, while the 'management' of the child in the dental situation falls to the dentist and his staff.)

Ideally, the parents should have been fully indoctrinated by the various dental health education methods into the modern ways of preventive dental care and are well prepared to look after the infant's teeth from the moment that they erupt into the mouth.

They are able to give the child a secure and caring background and to encourage it to explore new experiences from this safe base. There have been no unpleasant medical experiences or hospital admissions to colour the child's perception of the dental environment. Unfortunately these ideal conditions do not always apply!

First dental appointment

Although dental care and advice should always be available for mother and infant, the first formal dental appointment is usually arranged when the child is about 2 years old. Before that he may perhaps attend the surgery with other members of the family, older siblings or mother, for such pre-appointment visits allow him to become accustomed to the surroundings and the people.

Pre-appointment preparation

The first appointment for a young child must be planned carefully. It is important not to pick a time of day when he is getting tired or usually having a nap. The early morning is best when both the child and the dental team are freshest. In general, appointments should never be scheduled to last more than 20 minutes for 2 year olds, or 30–45 minutes for children over the age of 5 years, and some dentists prefer that the first appointment may be even shorter. A welcoming letter can be sent to the mother a few days before the appointment, confirming the date and time and including simple details of the importance of dental care, and what she may expect to happen at the first visit.

Before arriving at the surgery the mother should give the child a simple explanation of the visit such as 'going to see that nice man who wants to see how well we brush your teeth'. The child should wear ordinary clothes and not be dressed up specially, and if possible not have to make a long, tiring, complicated journey to and from the surgery.

The dental practice

The interface between the child's prior experience and the practice is where the dentist can begin to take more effective charge of the situation. He is in control of the surgery building, the staff who assist him and himself.

Reception

The waiting room should have a corner set aside for children, with suitable chairs and magazines and even a large 'can't be taken home' quiet toy or a rocking horse. A child should not be delayed in the waiting room for long but both child and parent will gain confidence from these outward signs that the practice is geared to meet children's needs. Some practices even have special children's sessions when the waiting room is entirely rearranged for smaller patients. This has the added bonus of children being able to see each other and also that the nervous adult patient does not have to listen to children's prattle. Many practices have a dental education room where the child can first meet and get used to the staff before reaching the dental chair. The case history may be taken there as well.

Dental surgery

It must be remembered that the dental surgery is to a great extent designed to make the dental surgeon feel at home, competent, and ready for anything and this does not necessarily conform with the child's perception of the ideal, safe place to be.

The dental team must be aware of the apprehensive child's heightened senses of sight, sound and smell. The surgery should be kept low key, quiet and well ventilated so that it doesn't smell strongly of antiseptics and solvents. As much of the equipment as possible should be kept hidden but easily accessible. The team should examine the surgery from a child's eye level from time to time to make sure that there are no frightening items on view that might seem to threaten the newcomer.

The dental team

The dentist must be careful about his choice of staff when preparing to treat children and select those who are able to demonstrate by their interest, appearance, knowledge and general demeanour that they are willing to take special care of each child patient. The mother is trusting the practice with a most precious member of the family and will be very sensitive to any possible slight. Particular attention should be paid to those responsible for reception duties, for the first contacts with the family both on the telephone, in writing and at the front door of the practice become most important indicators of the practice as a whole.

Dental surgeon

He must be sure that he really wants to treat young patients, for any lack of interest or confidence will quickly be read by both the child and the parent in this situation. He must be specially sensitive to the important part played by his appearance, facial expression, movements and above all the use of his voice.

The care procedure

Introducing the child to the dental environment

On arrival the receptionist should greet the child by his first name. The child and parent are then shown to the waiting room for a few minutes to take off outer clothes, and their mother can be encouraged to check if the child needs to go to the toilet. Every effort should be made not to keep them waiting for more than 10 minutes in the waiting room for that becomes part of the total appointment time as far as the child is concerned and he will tire more quickly when he finally reaches the surgery.

Should the parent accompany the child into the surgery? Some practitioners dislike having the parent present because they find it distracting, but on the whole there are many advantages to be gained. Their presence, particularly for the pre-school child, can be most reassuring. The mutually reacting triad of parent–child–dentist works well in building up a rapport, in gaining the parent's confidence as well as the child's in ensuring that there are no misunderstandings about the case history, in monitoring recent events and in gaining consent to treatment. The team must remember how much they depend upon the parent, who may well be feeling apprehensive, and always try to reassure them as well.

The dentist can decide the best place for the parent to sit in the surgery. Usually they should be encouraged to sit to one side of the room so that the child knows they are there, and given a magazine to read. For a small child they should sit where the child can actually see them. The parent (and the dental nurse) should be made to understand that it is best if they do not talk to the child while the dentist is undertaking treatment. The child needs to be able to concentrate on what the dentist is saying and becomes confused if others are giving him advice and encouragement as well, however well-meant.

In most cases, as the child grows older and more experienced he himself may find the parent's company in the surgery less welcome.

The dentist must beware when (a) both parents, (b) mother and grandmother, or (c) the parent of a teenager insist upon being present in the surgery, for in each case this is generally an early warning of impending poor cooperation from the patient.

Entering the surgery

First the child should be given a moment or two to become accustomed to the strange surroundings: the environment, the equipment and the dentist and his nurse.

Children tend to mirror the dentist's own reactions to them. They will look into his face and eyes and try to work out his intentions towards them. They will be affected by his tone of voice and body language. They are aware that kind-eyed people, who move slowly and deliberately and have low, slow voices do not mean harm. They appreciate it if the dentist knows their first name, or nickname—and pronounces it properly! The dentist should give them time to get to know and trust him and he must not appear to be in an impatient hurry.

Introduction to the care procedure

The child can be allowed to climb into the dental chair and get comfortable. Then the bib, the mouthwash, the lights, etc, can be slowly introduced while maintaining a fun approach. The dentist then commences taking the case history, remembering that the child is listening to everything that is said. Thus he must discourage long descriptions of previous bad behaviour ('he wouldn't open his mouth for the last dentist') for they can become a rehearsal for a repeat performance.

This 'getting to know you' period is an opportunity to assess the emotional climate of the family, the child's mental age, confidence, previous experience and likely cooperation.

The dentist proceeds through the stage of the gentle examination trying to show genuine affection, and no anger or impatience. Preferably he will use the well-known 'Tell, Show, Do' technique; e.g. Tell: 'I'm going to look at your teeth with a little mirror', Show: 'This little mirror here', Do: 'Open your mouth, let's see, good, well done!' The sequence is repeated as other instruments and procedures are introduced.

The dentist should praise the child's good behaviour and try to proceed quickly and efficiently. If possible, at the first appointment he should carry out some simple treatment procedure such as polishing the teeth with pleasant tasting toothpaste using the dental engine. The child can be warned about the sound that the engine or instrument will make, e.g. 'a cat purring' or 'an aeroplane' and thus encouraged to interpret the sensations as comfortable and pleasant, e.g. a 'tickle that will make your tooth laugh'. Some dentists explain unfamiliar equipment or activities in what has been called 'childrenese' of their own invention, e.g. high velocity suction = 'dentist's vacuum cleaner', tweezers = 'silver fingers', compressed air blast = 'a puff of wind'.

The treatment sequences can be planned over several appointments so that the child's escalating experience trains him to accept increasingly demanding procedures. It may be better to compromise by arranging short appointments confined to placing simple temporary restorations at an early stage before attempting more complex prolonged restorations.

The child's good behaviour should be rewarded with lots of praise and flattery.

The dentist should be alert to onset of signs of restlessness that indicate that the child is getting tired and that the session should be ended quickly. These include wriggling the feet and legs, lifting the head from the head rest frequently, ebbing cooperation and delaying tactics.

The session should end with a sense of achievement and friendly assurance. The dentist might discuss what will happen next time, but he must take care to leave nothing for the child's imagination to work on negatively.

As the child leaves he can be given some small token reward for good behaviour, e.g. badges, balloons, painting books, a 'go' on the computer game, etc.

Special cases

The very young child

This patient is likely to be apprehensive and afraid of new experiences and strangers. Keep him near his mother, letting her hold him on her knee in the dental chair. Talk to her first while he gets used to you. Proceed in an unhurried way. Try to gain the child's attention and interest. Praise some aspect of his appearance: his new shoes, the pattern on his shirt, the toy he is holding. Gently touch the child's hand, arm, shoulder, stroke his cheek—in sequence—don't appear to be in a hurry to examine his mouth!

Take care with your own voice, keep it low and slow and quiet. Use the child's first name. Get him to help by giving him something to hold such as a cotton-wool roll. Get him to open his mouth while you are some 5 to 6 feet away—then a closer look—then put on the

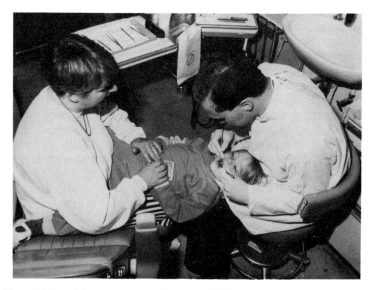

Figure 2.1 Examining an uncooperative young child

light 'because it's dark in there'—then find a mirror to examine him
and so on. Again use the 'Tell, Show, Do' sequence.

If this approach fails, keep calm and get mother to turn in the
chair so that her feet are on the floor and she is facing you. Adjust
your stool so that your lap is on the same level as hers. Ask the
mother to place the child so that its head is on your lap and its body
on hers. Ask her to control the child's legs under her elbows and its
hands with her hands (Figure 2.1). Stop the head rolling from side
to side with the heels of your hands. Use two mirrors or one and a
toothbrush handle. One handle is slipped between the child's back
teeth on one side as it opens its mouth to protest. Then you can
proceed with the examination and, using the alternate mirror handle
as a gag change sides as necessary. The procedure will be noisy but
you can clearly examine the mouth and teeth and even proceed as
far as gentle excavation of a cavity and dressing. Then sit the child
up 'to give its mother a good cuddle'. The child will understand and
forgive this mild restraint by its parent. However, it would not be
acceptable if the child was restrained on a stranger's knee instead
of its parent's for then a noisy encounter would lead to increased
separation anxiety for both parent and child.

The crying child

Children may cry in the dental surgery for a number of reasons;
Elsbach (1963) described the recognition of different kinds of crying
as diagnostic tool: Fear = a heart-rending wail; Pain = whimper;
Hurt = moan, groan; Rage = howl; Obstinate = a siren shriek;
Compensatory = grizzle, to drown the sound of the drill.

Preparing a child for an unpleasant procedure

(E.g. a dental extraction under local anaesthesia.) Tell him what
is to happen and why in simple terms, not too far in advance. Be
straightforward and choose your words carefully. Try to reduce
uncertainty. Don't resort to subterfuge: 'to lie like a dentist'! Take
care when discussing the case in front of him. Be prepared to
support the parent's anxieties, for they in turn can support the child,
but remove child from parent's influence if necessary, i.e. if their
reaction is not helping the child to remain calm.

At the time of operation, be firm, efficient, not unduly concerned
with emotional outbursts or crying. Give sympathetic help throughout. Don't minimize or exaggerate what is happening. Don't humili-
ate the emotional child, e.g. 'your little sister wouldn't cry like this'.
Try to get him to relax as much as possible. Distract his attention by

talking. An older child may have explained restraint applied to help him, e.g. holding someone's hand, or being held firmly by the parent.

Difficult children

Problems arise in providing dental care for children who are uncooperative and disruptive or for whom the perceived threat of entering the dental surgery precipitates bad behaviour.

In severe cases the parents and teachers have already noticed the moody, intense child who is slow to adapt to new experiences, The parents often suffer feelings of guilt, incompetence and anger. Instead of trying to help they want to transfer the blame for the child's actions to you: 'he's only like this at the dentist!'

The stubborn-resistant child

Usually caused by excessive scolding and punishment from unwise parents when it exhibited the normal behaviour patterns of child-hood and now it reacts to stress with stubbornness, back-talk and temper tantrums rather than crying.

The spoiled child

Arises from parental overprotection and overpermissiveness. The result can be a fearful, clinging, babyish or manipulating child playing on the inability of the parents to limit its behaviour and their desire to do everything for it at all times. This child can be a faddy eater with problems at mealtimes. It will also suffer severe separation anxiety, and endless other problems.

Changing such behaviours is mainly a learning process and demands consistency and limit-setting with a minimal emotional reaction of anger from you. On the occasions, and there will be some, when everything seems to be getting out of hand, you should resort to a 'time out' period where the child is sent out of the surgery for up to ten minutes to cool off before returning for a rapid conclusion of the appointment.

The anxious/fearful child

Although the real situation may be completely harmless and even beneficial, the individual's interpretation, plus the built-in innate fears and learned responses, take priority.

Consider how the mother, family and vicarious experience has prepared the child. Have siblings and school friends talked about 'needles, blood and drills'? Is the dentist perceived as a punishment?

Discover what first-hand dental experiences the child has already had. Some children's fear follows logically after an unwise or unpleasant experience in the dental chair. In many cases the child has been subjected to a prolonged treatment session too soon. Let the child know that you understand how it feels. Mentally 'put your arm around the child' and make it understand that you are on its side and that together you can tackle the dental problem.

Easy acceptance of dental care is best learned in a sequence of escalating steps of experience. If the steps are too great for a particular child it will be overwhelmed and become fearful. Try to modify your treatment plan accordingly.

Learn to be sensitive to the small signals of anxiety: in the eyes and face, which like the onset of restlessness indicate that a session should be ended quickly. Success in this respect means knowing when to stop.

Behaviour modification

Many behavioural problems, particularly those precipitated by fear and anxiety can be prevented or overcome by using the ideas expressed in the following sequences. They can serve to extinguish and desensitize existing fears. There is, however, no 'magic formula' for success every time.

1. Modelling: Encourage the child to base its behaviour on that of another good subject's example, e.g. watching siblings, friends, or even Teddy Bear enjoying dental treatment. Away from the surgery behaviour can be modelled by story books, TV tapes and slides about dental care, and by talks given to the parent and child before and after treatment.
2. Safe environment: Remember that all apprehensive children will have sharpened senses (sight, sound, smell, taste, touch) plus an active imagination, so try not to stimulate them unnecessarily. Be aware of the numerous basic fears that can be cued by the dental treatment situation and minimize them. Reduce the instruments on display. Keep the surgery quiet.
3. Pleasant activities: Plan your approach to emphasize the pleasant aspects of dentistry. Use the first visit, where possible, as a 'getting to know you' session in an unhurried yet short, morning appointment. Create good channels of communication with the child. Use its first name. Find some common interest outside the surgery—the child's pet, 'what are you missing at

school?', 'what did you get for your birthday?', etc. Get the child to relax. Always reward good behaviour verbally with immediate flattering praise and with a token, e.g. a sticker badge, at the end of the session.

4. Gradual introduction: Commence with simple treatment procedures using the 'Tell, Show, Do' technique. Develop a 'You and Me Together' rapport. Proceed to more demanding procedures by slow escalation. Praise and flatter a lot. Warn of the sounds that the instruments will make. Keep surgery quiet. Always avoid force and let the child have a sense of control.

Systematic desensitization (Gale and Ayer, 1969)

This has been used successfully to overcome dental phobia or extreme dental anxiety in older children and adults and may work by identifying items and gaining sympathetic understanding.

At a first session the therapist takes the patient's history and begins to teach him how to relax. At the next session the therapist helps the patient to construct a personal written hierarchy, setting the frightening things about dental treatment in order of intensity (e.g. 20 items: ranging from, say, (1) Thinking about going to the dentist. (2) Ringing up to make an appointment to see the dentist, to (20) The dentist is drilling my tooth.) By the third session the patient has learnt how to relax. Now and in further sessions the members of the hierarchy are presented from four to nine times with each visualization lasting from 15 to 45 seconds with an interval in between. In most cases the patient is desensitized after up to nine sessions and can start to accept dental treatment. The method is practical and flexible and enjoys a good success rate.

Pharmacological methods

In urgent cases treatment under sedation or a general anaesthetic may be indicated. Otherwise the dentist should not be tempted to use drugs too readily for routine care because although they may allow dental treatment to be done, their use will not solve the long-term behavioural problem.

Chapter 3

Diagnosis and treatment planning

History taking, diagnostic methods and treatment planning form the fundamental basis for the successful practice of children's dentistry. The manner in which they are carried out plays an important part in the establishment of good communication and rapport between the dental surgeon, the child and its parent, for it provides the opportunity to demonstrate the practitioner's care, skill and understanding of the parent and child's feelings and anxieties in ways that can do much to facilitate subsequent operative treatment.

Sometimes the preliminary meeting with the child can be arranged away from the dental chair and it may even be possible to take the initial history in a neutral area outside the surgery. Commonly, however, the procedure is carried out in the surgery, with the child in the dental chair or sitting on its parent's knee. In any case the history is best taken with the parent or responsible adult present to ensure accurate information, for example even the teenage child cannot be relied upon to give a full account of its medical history. Don't be in too much of a hurry at this stage, give the parent and child time to tell you things that are worrying them, and above all, *listen* to what is said and don't appear to be judgemental. *Think, be alert, be thorough.*

With practice a comprehensive system can be worked through quite quickly if the written record is kept short and to the point and does not include extensive reporting of pointless detail. Try to record the information in an orderly way.

Important facts (e.g. penicillin sensitivity) should be underlined or otherwise indicated in a prominent way (e.g. with a coloured sticker) on the front of the record card so that the operator is always alerted at later appointments.

History taking and examination

Personal Details

Name	**(? plus nickname)**
Address	**Telephone no.**
Age	**Date of birth**

Doctor's name, address and telephone no.
Referred by:

Date of examination

$C/O = complains\ of$ (put in patient's or parent's words)
  Chief complaint
  Other complaints
                    (in chronological order)

$M/H = Medical\ history$
  Is the child quite fit and well at present?
  Has the child been treated for a general illness during the last six months?
  Is the child taking any medicines or tablets?
  Has the child had the common childhood illnesses?
  Has the child ever had a serious illness?
  Has the child ever been in hospital and, if so, what for?
  Ask specifically if the child has ever had any heart or respiratory problems, rheumatic fever, blood disorders (e.g. anaemia or bleeding tendencies), jaundice, general allergies, or drug reactions (particularly to antibiotics or anaesthetics).
  At this stage it may be of value to ask if there were any problems in the antenatal–birth–infancy period that might throw light on subsequent growth and development.

$D/H = Dental\ history$
  Developmental history
  Eruption of teeth, dates, problems
  Infant feeding techniques/weaning
  Use of pacifier?
  Habits, e.g. thumbsucking
  Home dental hygiene care
  Diet history
  Fluorides—use of, including toothpaste
  Soft-tissue problems
  Toothache
  Past treatment and reaction to it (e.g. experience of LA and GA). Don't expand on any difficulties in front of the child or it will become a rehearsal for a repetition of the problem.

Family history
  Parents   Siblings
  Health of the family: may give clues to inherited disorders and to
     attitudes and behaviour
  Family diet

Social history
  Father's occupation
  School progress
  Contacts with other children

Clinical examination

(Follow the sequence:
1. OBSERVATION: Examine visually
2. PALPATION: Examine by touch
3. SPECIAL TESTS: Consider if further tests are needed)

General appraisal
Is the child well or ill, apathetic or alert, anxious or relaxed?
  Size   Weight   Stature
  Speech
  Gait
  Hands

Potential reaction to dental care
  Parent
  Child
     Intellect
     General behaviour
     Anxiety
Good response or management problem expected?

Head and neck
  Size and shape
  Facial symmetry—profile aesthetics
  Skin
  Hair
  Eyes—conjunctivae
  Ears

Extra-oral
  Main bony contours, jaws, TMJs
  Lips—lip posture
  Regional lymph glands

Intra-oral
Mucosa of vestibule, cheeks, sulcus, fraenum
Tongue, mucosa, movement
Floor of mouth
Hard and soft palate
Pharynx, tonsils
Salivary glands
Teeth: general eruptive state
    Number, form, size, structure, position,
    Orthodontic classification,
    Occlusion, Crowding, Spacing, Overjet, Overbite
Oral hygiene—general
Periodontal condition
Mobile teeth, tenderness to pressure
Denture or appliance
Saliva consistency

Chart of teeth
Recording decayed, missing and filled teeth, etc. This requires good
visual access (perhaps with magnification), a good light source and
the teeth should be dried, quadrant by quadrant. The teeth are
examined optically using a mouth mirror, touching the teeth gently
with a probe, checking the tooth surfaces systematically.

Provisional diagnosis

At this stage the information collected so far can be scrutinized and
in simple straightforward cases no further examination is required
to reach a diagnosis and form a treatment plan.

Other, more complex, cases require further thought and
investigation.

Surgical sieve

A systematic approach, such as that provided by the 'surgical sieve'
can be a good memory jogger and lead to further more specifically
aimed questions, tests and investigations to aid diagnosis.
    Is the disorder . . . ?
    Congenital
    Traumatic
    Infective—Acute or Chronic—Specific or Non-specific
    Neoplastic—Benign or Malignant
    Symptomatic (think through the main systems of the body)
    Obscure Cause

Special tests and investigations that may be considered

General
  Temperature, Pulse and Respiration Rates
  Height, Weight
Dental
  Pulp Tests: Thermal and Electrical
  Transillumination of teeth
  Radiographs (see below)
  Disclosing Solution
  Plaque Score
  Study Models, Photographs
  Diet Record
    (3 day record of all food and drink consumed—include one
    week-end day)
Laboratory
  Saliva Tests
  Haematology: Bleeding Time, Clotting Time, Haemoglobin,
    Differential Cell Count, Sickle-cell Test, etc.
  Immunology
  Microbiology
    Identify organisms and sensitivity
  Biopsy
  Urine analysis

Consultation

Letter to patient's doctor, Hospital department, etc. asking for
further information.

Firm diagnosis

Now interpretation of the results of the examination and tests and
any incoming information should lead to the arrival at a firm diagnosis upon which treatment can be planned. In some cases referral
for specialist advice or treatment may be indicated.

Treatment planning

Broadly, treatment and care plans fall into the following categories:

1. Home care.
2. Preventive and operative care in the dental surgery.
3. Monitoring future dental health.

Obviously, if the child is in pain or has an abscess, for example, the dentist should carry out the simplest and quickest emergency treatment to relieve it. Otherwise, where possible, it is better to complete a simple procedure successfully during a short early appointment before undertaking a more complex and time-consuming one to allow a dentally inexperienced child time to come to terms gradually with the sights, sounds, tastes and sensations of dental treatment. Similarly, the child should be introduced to local anaesthesia by a simple infiltration first, before attempting a nerve block.

A treatment plan for a child is never inflexible and dictatorial, and the priorities must be reviewed at each visit in order to take account of changes that can inevitably occur.

Consider:
Medical history
Behaviour management
Suitability for anaesthetic: LA, GA
Preventive treatment
    Caries control
        Prophylaxis
        OHI, Plaque control
        Diet counselling
        Fluoride
        Fissure Sealing
Operative treatment
    Restorations
Prosthetic treatment
    Extractions/Surgery
Orthodontic treatment
Drugs to be prescribed
DISCUSS THE TREATMENT PLAN WITH THE PARENT TO GAIN CONSENT BEFORE PROCEEDING.

Example of forming a treatment plan

First appointment
Limited to Case History and Examination plus bite-wing radiographs ('Getting to know you' session).
Relevant details:
    John Example, aged 7. New to the practice.
    C/O No complaints.
    Medical History
    Cardiac Murmur. Recently examined by Dr B. Medic at General Hospital: Case No BZ1234.

Dental History
  Extraction of two primary molars at dental hospital at age 5.
  Under general anaesthetic without antibiotic cover as far as
  mother can remember.
Family History
  Mother already attends the practice. Has high caries rate herself.
Potential Reaction
  Caring mother
  Apprehensive child
Findings: Minimal occlusal caries in upper right first permanent
  molar. Poor oral hygiene.

Treatment Plan

1. Write to Dr Medic at General Hospital.
2. Delay routine dental care until a reply has been received.
3. Then make an early morning appointment as soon as possible.
    To bring toothbrush next time.
4. Meanwhile mother asked to complete a diet record form.
5. Arrange dental health education session.
6. Slow introduction to dental treatment.
7. Restore carious tooth and fissure seal other permanent molars.
8. Put child on the recall list for 4-monthly check-up.

Letter to Dr B. Medic, General Hospital.
Dear Dr Medic,
re John Example, Date of Birth
Patient's Address
General Hospital Number: BZ1234
This 7-year-old boy is now attending this practice for dental
treatment and when I examined him on (date) I found that he
needed a filling under local anaesthesia and to have his teeth cleaned
and polished. I understand that he is under your care for his heart
condition and I would be grateful to have your advice with regard
his fitness to receive the proposed dental treatment and your
recommendations about antibiotic cover.
Yours sincerely,

Reply: (Letter placed in patient's notes) John Example has an
innocent heart murmur and does not require antibiotic cover for
dental treatment. Fit for local anaesthetic.

Second appointment
Dental health education session for mother and child together.
Opportunity to explain about home care with regard to diet (check
the diet record information which the mother has collected), use of
fluorides, oral hygiene, plaque disclosure, tooth brushing. Mother
to be shown how to brush John's teeth. Mother also to be given
educational pamphlets, fluoride tablets if appropriate, and disclosing tablets. Every effort will be made to build up John's confidence and gain a good rapport with him. Treatment needs for next
appointments to be explained.

Third appointment
Introduction to dental procedures. Teeth polished with a rubber
cup. (John now responding well.)

Fourth appointment
Upper right first permanent molar to be restored under local
anaesthesia. Remaining permanent molars to be fissure sealed. (If
John had not been responding well this may have been done before
the restoration was attempted at a fifth appointment.) Follow-up
appointment to review condition in four months' time.

Future care will include regular dental check-ups: updating
information about John's general health, monitoring his diet, oral
hygiene and dental condition, maintaining a good rapport with
John and his mother. From his previous history it will be important
to consider further fissure sealing as the second permanent molars
erupt, to remain alert for onset and treatment of further dental
caries and for orthodontic problems arising as a result of the
premature extraction of primary teeth.

Radiographic examination

Because of the genetic and somatic effects of ionizing radiation it is
important to keep radiographic exposure of any patients, especially
children, to a minimum. Radiographs should not be taken
routinely, but only when clinically required. Always ask about
previous radiographs that have been taken, both for dental and
other reasons and try to defer further cumulative X-ray exposure
where possible. Children under the age of 5 should rarely need
dental radiographs.

Protective lead aprons should be used to protect the child's
thyroid and gonad areas during X-ray exposure. A thyroid shield
collar may also be used where it does not impede the X-ray beam.

Extra-fast films are recommended to reduce exposure times.

Rehearse the film-taking procedure using the 'Tell, Show, Do' sequence to check that the child can cooperate. Choose the least difficult radiographic technique that will give an adequate image. To avoid unnecessary delay have the X-ray machine set and ready before positioning the film.

Where a child is handicapped or not sufficiently cooperative to sit still while the film is being exposed it may be necessary for them to sit on their parent's knee for they can help to support the head. Under these circumstances it is most important to protect the adult with a radiation protective apron, plus a protective glove if the film is to be hand held. If the mother is pregnant or there is a possibility that she might be then the procedure must be postponed until another member of the child's family is available to support the child.

Radiographs might be considered for:

Investigation of pain.

Investigation following trauma to the teeth and jaws.

Investigation of swellings or tumours.

Checking for the presence of interproximal caries.

Deep caries.

Root canal therapy.

Orthodontic diagnosis.

Choice of radiographs that might be taken for a child:

1.	Periapical	Use a small child-size film because of lack of space, e.g. the shallow palate
2.	Bite-wing	Use a small film with its long axis at right angles to the occlusal plane. This will allow the apices of the primary molars to be seen on the radiograph
3.	Occlusal	
4.	Lateral oblique	Where intra-oral film refused
5.	Orthopantomogram	General view to monitor mandible, maxilla and all teeth present, both erupted and unerupted
6.	Lateral skull	Cephalometry
7.	Occipito-mental	Facial bones and antra
8.	Postero-anterior	Skull, facial bones, temporomandibular joints.

Chapter 4

Preventive dentistry

The World Health Organisation in Geneva has done much to energize and coordinate the international approach to the study of dental disease by introducing definitions, epidemiological standards and guideline advice with regard to the strategies of initiating dental treatment. The following is based to a certain extent upon the WHO concepts.

Definitions

Preventive dentistry: procedures or courses of action which prevent the onset of dental disease.

1. *Primary prevention.* Preventing the onset of disease:
    (a) Health education to improve oral hygiene.
    (b) Nutrition programmes to raise standards of nutrition and diet.
    (c) Periodic dental inspections to enable early detection of any dental disease.

2. *Secondary prevention.* Slowing the process of disease:
    (a) Treatment of early signs of disease to prevent progression.
    (b) Screening and recall examinations.

3. *Tertiary prevention.* Rehabilitation:
    (a) Treatment by restoration.
    (b) Controlling established periodontal disease.

The *incidence* of a disease indicates the number of occurrences of that disease over a stated period of time.

The *prevalence* of a disease refers to the number of cases in a population at a particular instant.

Background

Preventive dentistry has good prospects in young patients. The two most important aspects are the prevention of dental caries and periodontal disease.

Current surveys show two major trends in world oral health status:

1. Deterioration for most of the developing countries with high periodontal disease prevalence and dental caries prevalence continuing to increase.
2. Improvement for most of the highly industrialized countries with reductions of dental caries prevalence and indications that periodontal disease prevalence may be falling.

During recent decades there have been many reports about the decreasing prevalence of dental caries in children in the UK. This is thought to be due to the combined effects of a reduced consumption of sugary foods, the widespread use of fluoride tooth paste, water fluoridation schemes, the action of supplemental fluoride tablets and drops and the application of topical fluoride in dental surgeries (generally reserved for children with a high caries activity or the handicapped).

As a result there has been a reduction of dental caries, as designated by DMFS scores for example, of 30% to 50% in the last two decades.

However, in spite of this improvement, in 1990 it was estimated that in the UK 50% of 5-year-old children had active decay in their primary teeth and one-third of older children had untreated decay in permanent teeth (British Paedodontic Society, 1990). Although the mean experience has fallen there are still groups of children to be found who have a higher caries incidence than average. For example, this may be found in handicapped children, or those living in inner cities, or children of first generation immigrants from developing countries, whose rising standard of living leads to increased sugar intake and a large caries incidence. Thus it is constantly important to define, predict and identify priority target populations.

Health education

Any combination of learning opportunities and teaching activities designed to facilitate voluntary adaptations of behaviour that are conducive to health.

Objectives of dental health education

To influence dental knowledge and behaviour in an effective and cost-efficient way.

Knowledge: The well-educated know:

1. That teeth are important for masticating efficiency, appearance and speech.
2. That dental disease is preventable and with proper care teeth should last for life.
3. The fundamental knowledge of the relationship:
   (a) between sucrose in the diet and dental caries.
   (b) between good oral cleanliness and periodontal disease.

Behaviour: Motivated behaviour will mean that the individuals will:

1. Reduce their sucrose intake in the diet.
2. Clean their mouths effectively.
3. Attend regularly for appropriate dental check-ups as recommended by the dental services.

Where children are concerned objectives can be focused more precisely towards specific age groups.

Age 0–5

1. The parent's knowledge and motivation must be emphasized so that their example and actions will affect the young child.
2. The parents and grandparents, teachers and others should be made aware of the dangers to the child's teeth of sugar in drinks, food, confectionery, etc. The child should be weaned from the bottle by the age of 1 year. Confectionery as a love token or reward should be discouraged and substitutes suggested, such as small toys.
3. The child should see the example of its parents and siblings brushing their own teeth. The parent should clean the child's teeth twice a day, after breakfast and last thing before bed-time.
4. From now until the age of 12 years the use of fluoride supplements should be considered in accordance with local professional advice based on water fluoride levels.

Age 6–10

1. The child should be fully educated about the importance of its teeth and motivated about diet choices and oral hygiene. It must know about safe diet items.
2. The child should be taught the best methods of oral hygiene in its own individual case, using a fluoride toothpaste and shown the use of disclosing agents.
3. The child should have regular dental check-ups without anxiety or fear to initiate early preventive action in the case of incipient

caries or periodontal disease and to monitor growth and development and the possible need for orthodontic advice and treatment.

Age 11 plus

1. Attitudes and beliefs should be regularly monitored, revised and updated during dental check-ups.
2. In the early teens there may be a tendency for boys to fail to keep check-up appointments. All teenagers tend to discount previous good advice and follow the food and drink fads or fashions of their peers. It takes a particularly tactful and vigilant approach by health carers to avoid a period of neglect.
3. At this age the social importance of appearance and fresh breath become important motivants.

Methods of health education

The objective of health education is to affect people's attitudes and beliefs with regard to dental health so that they appreciate the value of their dental structures and are motivated to take care of them by effective means. This involves using the most effective means of communication available so that the target audience will understand, believe, remember and act upon the information being transferred. It requires a great deal of careful thought and preparation to overcome the barriers of apathy and lack of attention where the recipient does not listen, does not understand and does not care.

Education may be aimed at different kinds of targets:

1. Mass. The general public.
2. Community. Local groups.
3. Small Groups.
4. Individuals. One to one.

Mass
The message has to be simple and universal. No adjustment can be made for individual circumstances or condition. The mass media of film, TV, radio, press, etc. are used. This method is financially expensive and its effects are difficult to assess. If the message is repeated too often it tends to get lost by familiarity and may have limited long-term impact.

Community
Now the message can be aimed a little more precisely and can take

into account the local life-style, dialects, language, and financial status. From the start the actual requirements of the smaller community may be sampled and assessed and there is the possibility of checking the effect of a community campaign. Setting up the campaign may involve the use of a work force including local Health Education Officers, Health Visitors, Doctors, Nursing Staff, Teachers and Social Workers as well as Dentists and Dental Auxiliaries. Again the mass media may be used but concentrating on local broadcasting programming etc. Poster campaigns on local hoardings, buses, stations, etc. can be considered. Local campaigns last for a finite period or again over-familiary may produce apathy.

Groups
Here the educational effectiveness improves dramatically. The target groups of mothers or schoolchildren, etc. are more homogeneous and together in one place. They are likely to be of similar age, experience, social status and ethnic background. They are present under the eye of the educator who can plan a presentation specifically for them and adapt it to make allowances for audience reaction. To be most effective the presenter herself should not be far from the status of the audience. (A presentation given by a famous football player or TV star may bring too loud and distracting a personality to the group for them to hear the message clearly.) The educator is available to answer questions, lead a group discussion, and test the audience's understanding. The presentation will be helped by the inclusion of slides, videos, films, posters, pamphlets, etc. (all of which can be obtained from voluntary bodies, commercial organizations, the General Dental Council Charitable Trust or the Health Education Authority. See Appendix B: Sources.)

Individuals
The one-to-one teaching arrangement seems an effective and readily monitored method. The educator has the chance to concentrate upon the specific individual. He can see if the subject is responding, or conversely getting bored and restless, and can immediately adapt the communication line accordingly. Again the communication media can be useful but now the child can become more actively involved in practical demonstrations of, for example, oral hygiene techniques on models and in his own mouth. The educator may be an oral hygienist, dental therapist or the dental surgeon himself. The tuition may take place in the dental surgery or in a special dental education room with a mirror and a sink.

Home care/self care

The motivated individual or parent should be concerned about four main areas of dental health care:

1. Diet.
2. Oral hygiene/plaque control.
3. Fluorides.
4. Regular check-ups.

1. Diet

Control of cariogenic diets. Studies support the view that caries can develop only in the presence of sugars, both natural sucrose, fructose and glucose (in fruit and vegetables) and other highly refined carbohydrates, especially sucrose. Caries is more directly related to the frequency of consuming sugary foods and drinks and the time taken for oral clearance than to the total consumption. All natural fruit juices have a very high sugar content as do most fizzy drinks; they also present the additional hazard of a low (acid) pH. Parents and older children themselves should try to make an informed choice of foods and food products that are low in sugar content and try to eliminate those with high sugar content from the family and snack diet. (Food sugar content lists are available such as the one in *Which* magazine, Nov. 1987, and from the Health Education Authority.)

Examples:

	Teaspoonfuls of sugar
Chocolate digestive biscuit (one)	1
Cola drink (330 ml)	7
Fruit yoghurt (150 g)	5
Milk chocolate (small bar 50 g)	5
Chocolate caramel bar (65 g)	8

Sugar is also listed in the contents of tinned baked beans, tomato ketchup and sweet pickle, etc.

Babies should not be got off to sleep with a propped bottle or given reservoir comforters. They should be weaned off the bottle by the age of 1 year to avoid inevitable 'feeding bottle caries'. Delayed weaning from the breast will also cause dental caries when feeding on demand.

Children should be given satisfying well-balanced meals so that they do not need to supplement them with snack food and drinks in between. They should be brought up to avoid consumption of sweets and confectionery except occasionally at mealtimes.

Teenagers must be careful not to lapse into popular junk food fads as these are often sweet or contain hidden sugar even when savoury.

2. Oral hygiene/plaque control

Self-performed oral hygiene with non-fluoride dentifrices has been shown to be an ineffective way of preventing dental caries. However, toothbrushing for caries control is effective when fluoride toothpaste is used and this must be at least once daily, although the effect improves if the teeth are brushed with paste twice a day. Children under the age of 5 years tend to swallow toothpaste and the amount placed on the brush each time must be carefully limited, generally to a 'pea-sized' quantity. A lot of effort is needed to get older children to brush effectively. Nevertheless, the importance of oral hygiene in the control of periodontal disease means that educational programmes to encourage toothbrushing are worthwhile.

Equipment
Toothbrush of appropriate size (the Health Education Authority recommends nylon, multitufted brushes with, for children a 20 mm × 10 mm head, and for adults a 22–28 mm × 10–13 mm head), fluoride toothpaste, dental floss for interdental cleaning of the permanent teeth, disclosing agents, mirror (mouth mirror), light source, water, sink.

The very young child must have its teeth brushed by its parent at least once a day, but preferably after breakfast and last thing at night before bed. This may best be achieved with the child standing with its back to the seated adult who can look down over the child's head while brushing the teeth. As the child gets older it will start to attempt this oral hygiene for itself but will still need the additional help and supervision of an adult. Children need every encouragement in order to get them into the habit of brushing their teeth every day. No specific method of brushing is best in the primary and mixed dentition. Disclosing solutions and tablets are valuable aids for self-evaluation and self-instruction in older children.

3. Fluorides

The parent should follow local professional advice about fluoride supplements for children, and understand its importance in everyday oral hygiene procedures.

4. Regular check-ups

The parent must ensure that the children attend for regular dental check-ups as recommended by the local dental services. She may have to initiate the first dental appointment herself when the child reaches 2 years of age.

Prevention in the dental surgery

1. Regular check-ups

(a) Initiate an efficient recall system.
(b) Time the check-up appointments appropriately, i.e. more frequently for children with a high caries rate and low motivation for self-care. Initially it is best to recall all children at 4-monthly intervals until the dentist is familar with their needs, predicted caries and motivation.

Check-ups are necessary to:
(a) Monitor self-care.
(b) Monitor growth and development, caries, periodontal condition, etc.
(c) Maintain rapport with the child and reduce fear and anxiety.

Note: The dentist may be first to detect general disease in the course of these regular monitoring checks.

2. Prevention instruction

Educators
Dentist, Dental Surgery Assistant, Oral Hygienist, Health Educator, Dental Therapist.

One to one, in the surgery or the education room.
Teaching aids: videos, models, giant toothbrushes, computer games, samples, posters, pamphlets etc., mirrors and sink.

Primary instruction in self-applied preventive methods requires subsequent support and monitoring through periodic professional examinations, during which the dentist will diagnose any disorders that may have developed, assess the effectiveness of the patient's control measures and give or arrange for further instructions and encouragement.

Diet analysis
In the case of the caries-prone child it is helpful to check on a child's diet for caries-promoting items by getting the parent, or the older

child himself, to write down everything that the child eats or drinks over a two-day period, including one week-end day (Saturday or Sunday, when most families may eat a holiday diet). The list should include the times and amounts of consumption. Subsequently the educator can analyse the list with the parent and child and point out any items that are likely to affect the child's dental health. Positive guidance is required.

3. Operator-applied preventive measures

(a) Prophylaxis. The child's teeth can be cleaned thoroughly using the dental engine.
(b) Topical application of fluorides (see below).
(c) Fissure sealing.

Fluorides and dental caries

1. When fluoride is incorporated into dental enamel during tooth development it produces an enamel crystalline structure more resistant to acid and may reduce the fissure depth.
2. Any fluoride present in the oral environment reduces the metabolism of sugars by bacteria thus cutting down acid production and plaque growth.
3. The presence of fluoride in plaque enhances natural salivary remineralization or 'repair' of early carious enamel lesions or 'white spots' by reprecipitation of enamel crystals.

Systemic and topical fluorides

Water fluoridation

Fluoridation of public water supplies involves the adjustment of existing fluoride concentration to an optimum depending on local climate and thus daily water consumption. For those living in a fluoridated area it confers a reduced prevalence and severity of dental caries in childhood which continues into adult life.

Concentration	Reduction in tooth decay (from an initially high rate)
0.7–1.2 mg/l	50–65%

The fluoride ion level of the water supply in a particular area can be readily found out by contacting the District Dental Officer, the local

Water Company or the Water Board Authority such as the ones on the following list.

Anglian Water Authority	0480 433433
Central Scotland Water Authority	0786 62811
Lothian Regional Council	0312 299292
North West Water Authority	0925 724321
Northumbrian Water Authority	0912 843151
Severn Trent Water Authority	0217 224000
South West Water plc	0392 219666
Southern Water plc	0903 205252
Strathclyde Regional Council	0412 273409
Thames Water Authority	071 837 3300
Welsh Water Authority	0874 3181
Wessex Water Authority	0272 290611
Yorkshire Water plc	0532 448201

Fluoride supplements: fluoride tablets and drops

Where the drinking water is deficient in fluoride benefits of the same order can be obtained by the daily ingestion of fluoride supplements starting with drops at age 6 months changing to tablets for the older child until age 12 (when the second molar erupts). This requires regular daily consumption supervised by a dedicated parent.

Recommended daily fluoride supplement
(Given as fluoride tablets or drops)

6 months to 2 years	0.25 mg F
2 to 4 years	0.50 mg F
4 to 12 years	1.00 mg F

In areas where the water supply contains 0.3–0.7 mg/l doses should be halved, and where it is 0.7 mg/l and over no supplement is needed.

Allowing the tablets to dissolve in the mouth gives an additional topical effect.

Topical fluoride

Fluoride toothpastes
These can be recommended everywhere except for young children living in areas of known endemic fluorosis. The incidence of new carious lesions can be reduced by 20–30% though this may be even better over prolonged usage. Currently toothpastes sold in the UK contain up to 1450 ppm of fluoride.

Mouth-rinsing with dilute fluoride solutions
Supervised mouth-rinsing has been shown to reduce dental decay by about 35% when used daily (0.5 g/l sodium fluoride containing 225 ppm fluoride), weekly or fortnightly (2 g/l solution). Weekly is most practicable.

Operator-applied fluoride compounds
Gels, solutions and varnishes have been tested and accepted in various degrees. Regular professional application is time-consuming and expensive and may only be of practical use for special groups, e.g. the medically compromised, and in cases of high caries activity.

Acidulated phosphate fluoride (APF) agents can contain up to 12 000 ppm fluoride. In young children the plasma levels of fluoride have been found to be unacceptably high, from orally retained gel, after the application of fluoride gels in trays (Lecompte, 1987).

Duraphat fluoride varnish contains 23 000 ppm fluoride and must be used carefully and in limited amounts. If the child is already taking fluoride tablets it should not take a tablet on the day that the varnish or other high fluoride level agent has been applied in the surgery.

Problems with fluorides
It is important to monitor and control the intake of fluoride. If excessive amounts of fluoride agents are ingested they can cause enamel hypoplasia, mottled enamel or even poisoning.

Beware of the over-enthusiastic parent who wants to give their child extra fluoride for extra protection. Make your advice about fluoride very clear and simple and make sure it is understood and followed properly.

1. Ingestion of excess fluoride from any source under the age of 6 years may result in visible white patches on the anterior permanent teeth when they erupt.
2. The parent must supervise the child's tooth brushing. They should allow no more than a 'pea-size' quantity of fluoride tooth paste on the brush each time and make sure the bulk of it is spat out again after brushing and not swallowed.
3. Fluoride mouthwashes must be used under supervision, must not be swallowed, and are not suitable for children under the age of 8 years.
4. Check the fluoride regime for sick children very carefully, especially if they are underweight.

Acute toxicity of fluoride—see Chapter 11

Fissure sealants

Pit and fissure sealants are plastics applied to the occlusal surfaces of posterior teeth by a simple acid-etch method to prevent dental caries. Sealants can also prevent early carious lesions from developing further. They are valuable because, while fluoride is more effective in preventing smooth-surface caries, sealants protect pits and fissures. They provide a simple method of treating early carious lesions as an alternative to amalgam or other restorations which require tooth tissue loss during cavity preparation.

Sealant resins may be filled or unfilled, self-curing or light-cured, colourless or tinted. Their successful application demands the maintenance of a dry field and a carefully timed, meticulous technique following the manufacturer's instructions wtih precision. Even though a tooth has been sealed it should be reviewed regularly and included in routine bite-wing radiographic checks.

The following clinical guidelines for the use of fissure sealants have been recommended (British Paedodontic Society, Policy Document, 1987):

Patient selection for fissure sealing
Children with special needs (medically compromised, mentally or physically handicapped, or from a disadvantaged social background), and children with a history of extensive caries in their primary teeth should have all first permanent molars sealed as soon as clinically possible after their eruption. Children who had caries-free primary dentitions should be monitored regularly.

Tooth selection for fissure sealing
The technique is most effective when used on the occlusal surfaces of permanent molar teeth. The sealing of primary molars is not normally advised. Sealants should be applied as soon as it is clinically possible to gain moisture control, and certainly within two years of eruption. Any child with occlusal caries in one first molar should have the fissures of the remaining sound first permanent molars sealed. Occlusal caries affecting first permanent molars indicates a need to seal the second permanent molars as soon as they erupt (Worthington *et al.*, 1988). Teeth to be sealed should be free of approximal caries.

Clinical circumstances
Teeth with doubtful occlusal fissures should be examined with bite-wing radiographs in order to estimate the extent of the lesion and to ensure that it has not led to 'occult' or 'mushroom' caries

(see Chapter 13). If dentine involvement cannot be seen radiographically, the fissure should be sealed as a preventive measure and kept under close review.

Fissure sealants are used in conjunction with preventive resin fillings (see Chapter 6).

Method of fissure sealing
The technique broadly follows the same sequence, but precise details of mixing, setting time, etc. must be checked in the manufacturer's instructions for the particular material chosen.

1. Carry out a prophylaxis on the whole occlusal surface using an oil-free, non-fluoride polishing paste. Wash the tooth thoroughly with a water spray. Rake along the fissures with a probe to loosen or remove any trapped paste or other debris and wash the tooth thoroughly once more. Such prophylaxis is generally recommended by the manufacturers although it has been shown that there is no significant difference in sealant retention if it is not carried out (Donnan and Ball, 1988).
2. Isolate the quadrant carefully with cotton wool rolls or rubber dam and blow the tooth dry with an air syringe for 30 sec. (Beware of a compressed air source that is contaminated with oil or moisture: from time to time check that the output from the air syringe is clean and dry by blowing on a cool glass slab.)
3. Apply the etchant solution or gel to the occlusal surface of the tooth, and any other surfaces to be sealed, for the recommended time (usually 60 sec). Don't scrub the surfaces with the applicator for this will remove the etched surface as it is formed. Then rinse the areas thoroughly, first with a water jet and then with an air and water spray from a 3 in 1 syringe, for at least 30 sec. Control the water in the mouth with a vacuum tip. Dry the surfaces with the air syringe once more. The etched surfaces should appear frosty and opaque, if not, re-etch for a further 20 sec.
4. Change the wet cotton wool rolls for fresh ones. Do not allow the etched surfaces to be contaminated with saliva. Again blow the etched surfaces dry. From now on a dry field is essential.
5. Mix the self-curing sealant components carefully to avoid the incorporation of air bubbles. Follow the manufacturer's instructions exactly with regard to mixing, placing and setting times. Light-cured agents are ready-mixed.
6. Apply the sealant to the fissures with the disposable applicator or brush supplied. Allow chemically activated materials the appropriate time to set and confirm this by testing the remainder left in the mixing vessel. The outer surface of set

sealant, in contact with air, remains unpolymerized. All surfaces sealed with light-cured materials must be given a full 60 sec exposure to the curing light and the light tip must not be allowed to touch the setting sealant and become attached to it.

7. Wipe the surface of the set sealant with a cotton wool roll and check with a probe for coverage and retention. Remove the isolation materials, allow the patient to rinse the taste away and then check the occlusion. Where necessary use articulating paper and adjust the occlusion by grinding surplus sealant away with a small stone or diamond instrument in a slow handpiece.

8. Review the sealed teeth at six-monthly intervals to ensure that the sealant is intact and not leaking. If a sealant fails check the margins carefully to ensure that the fissure remains caries free before re-etching the tooth and adding further sealant. In cases of doubt consider placing a preventive resin restoration.

Chapter 5

Control of pain and anxiety

Local anaesthesia

The use of local anaesthesia plays a most important part in the provision of painless dental treatment and does much to reduce and prevent a child's fear and anxiety. However, it is not a substitute for gentle handling, for as Roberts and Sowray (1987) point out, the local anaesthetic agent only produces local analgesia and thus the child remains aware of every other aspect of the treatment procedure and still needs the care and support of the operator.

Some experienced operators may be able to decide when a procedure can be carried out without causing any discomfort, but it is always better to err towards using local anaesthesia to ensure that the child never experiences pain due operative treatment.

Local anaesthetic agents

(a) For injection
Lignocaine HCl 2% and Adrenaline 1/80 000 (Xylocaine injection 2% with adrenaline (Astra)). This preparation is considered to be universally safe and effective.

Prilocaine HCl 3% and Felypressin 0.03 units/ml (Citanest 3% with Octapressin (Astra)). This is generally reserved for patients who have cardiac rhythm problems and where there is a risk of inadvertent intravenous administration.

Both are available in cartridges for use in dental syringes, with or without self-aspiration. Their effect lasts for just over an hour.

(b) For surface anaesthesia
Lignocaine HCl 5% in a water-miscible base (Xylocaine ointment (Astra)).

Needles

(a) For infiltration: 30 gauge ¾ inch (0.3 × 19 mm).
(b) For nerve blocks: 27 gauge 1⅜ inch (0.4 × 34 mm).

Preliminaries

Always check the child's medical history to make sure that there is
no contraindication to the drug injection.

Never inject into inflamed tissues or near discharging sinuses for
not only will this fail to anaesthetize the area adequately but it will
also spread the infection.

The child's first experience of having local anaesthesia is very
important because a successful outcome paves the way to an easy
acceptance of dental injections in the future. Nevertheless, give
every injection as carefully as the first.

Ideally you will have developed a good rapport with the child so
that you are mutually confident. Don't attempt injections for a
young child who is tired, restless and not listening to you.

If possible choose to give an infiltration injection in the upper jaw
as an introduction, because they are usually successful, do not
require deep needle penetration, and they do not anaesthetize large
areas of tissue, which the inexperienced child may find upsetting.
If possible choose a simple speedy operation after the introductory
injection has been given.

Explanation

Tell the child what is about to happen. Explain in simple words,
appropriate to the child's age, choosing them carefully so that they
do not evoke fear. Use terms like 'putting the tooth to sleep', 'sleepy
water', 'a scratch', 'a pinch', 'going numb', 'funny tingly feeling',
'fat lip', etc.

Preparation

Have your dental surgery assistant present alongside the chair to
assist in passing the prepared syringe, etc.

Continue to control the child by your voice and non-verbal
gestures. Any tendency for the child to make sudden movements can
be hampered by an all-enveloping dental bib and by getting the
child to 'hold nurse's hand'.

Take up some surface anaesthetic ointment on the end of a cotton
wool roll or cotton bud. Use the other end of the roll or bud to
dry the mucosa in the area of injection and then, reversing the

applicator, apply the surface anaesthetic to the injection sites. Hold the applicator in position for a minute to allow the agent to work properly. A saliva ejector may be required. Keep talking slowly, in a low confidential manner, about distracting things such as pets, TV programmes, etc., but not subjects that require a response. Tiny children can be told a simple story.

Injection

Try to keep the syringe out of sight. Tell the child to sit still. Remove the cotton applicator from the mouth keeping one finger in place holding the lip away from the injection site. Receive the prepared syringe from the dental surgery assistant, needle guard already removed, passed to you from low down, out of the child's view. Bring the syringe up to the side of the mouth and while continuing to talk to distract the child, convey the needle tip to the injection site and commence the injection, still talking in a calm tone. Always proceed in a slow, purposeful manner (Figure 5.1).

Inject very slowly and deliberately and when the full amount required has been delivered pass the syringe back out of sight to the dental surgery assistant who will collect it in a dish. (Beware of needle stick injuries!) Now get the child to move around after sitting

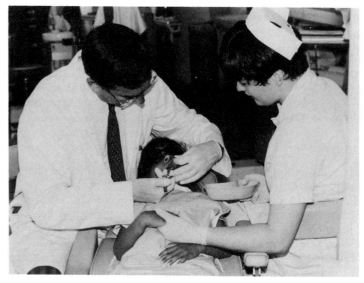

Figure 5.1 Child receiving a local anaesthetic injection

still so well. Get him to rinse out. Begin to explain again what he should be feeling at the injection site. Stay with him at this moment, for although the operator feels more relaxed now that he has succeeded in giving the injection, the child, suddenly losing the feeling from part of his mouth and lips, can begin to feel very alarmed. Stay alongside and continue to reassure him. If possible show him his face in a large mirror to confirm that all is still there and well. Don't be in too much of a hurry to continue. Wait until you are sure that the local anaesthetic agent has worked before you commence potentially painful treatment.

Types of injections

1. Infiltration

Anaesthesia of all primary teeth, upper and lower, can be achieved by infiltration injections. This is because, in the child, the buccal and labial bone is thin and there are more vascular bone perforations which allow the solution to reach the apices of the teeth. However, the success rate has to be qualified in the case of the mandibular second primary molar for the child over the age of 5 years when the bone in this region begins to grow denser (Wright et al., 1987). The technique is also used in the permanent dentition for all the maxillary teeth and the mandibular incisors and canines.

The injection is given at the reflection of the labial/buccal mucosa with the alveolus, with the syringe held parallel to the long axis of the upper teeth. The mucosa is stretched and pulled onto the needle which is then advanced, after injecting a few drops of solution, towards the periosteum. Try to avoid contacting bone if possible because this can cause after-pain; if you do contact bone withdraw the syringe slightly before continuing the injection. One ml of the agent is injected slowly taking at least 30 sec. It is not necessary to administer a full 2 ml cartridge for a child. A further few drops will be needed lingually or palatally for extractions or the application of rubber dam clamps or matrices.

2. Intra-papillary

Here the point of injection is into the sound, healthy interdental papilla in the primary dentition, distal to the tooth to be anaesthetized. This injection is not recommended if the gingival condition is poor. Start the injection, wait until the area is affected by the anaesthetic agent and then move the needle more deeply through the interdental space and inject the palatal or lingual mucosa as well. Anaesthesia is thus obtained with only one injection. This technique does not require the administration of a large volume of local anaesthetic solution. There may be some degree of after-pain when the injection wears off.

3. Inferior dental block

This technique is used to anaesthetize the mandibular molar teeth and adjacent tissues.

It is very important to use aspirating syringes for these deep injections in children for they are particularly vulnerable to the

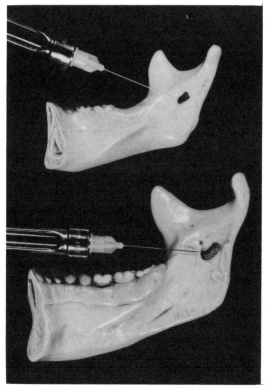

Figure 5.2 The angle of the inferior dental block injection must take into account the changing anatomy of the growing mandible at different ages

complication of intravascular injection, which can lead to systemic action of the vasoconstrictor drugs and cause fainting and collapse. The injection is usually given with a 27 gauge needle.

Care must be taken to establish the local anatomy of the mandible: the angle of the mandible in a child is more obtuse than in the adult (Figure 5.2) and the area needs to be palpated and visualized carefully to find the correct anatomical landmarks. The mandibular foramen is at the same height as the occlusal plane of the primary teeth.

The operator should place his thumb in the buccal sulcus sliding it back over the buccinator and into the retromolar fossa, palpating the anterior border of the ascending ramus of the mandible. His first and second fingers should grip the mandible to palpate the anatomical shape accurately and to steady the jaw. The injection is to be deposited where the inferior dental nerve bundle enters the lingual foramen on the ascending ramus of the mandible. This target now lies at a point at the centre of the triangle formed by the tips of the thumb and first two fingers. The needle will enter the mucosa at the level of the midline of the thumbnail. The needle passes through the buccinator lateral to its attachment to the pterygomandibular raphé, with the barrel of the syringe over the premolar or primary molar region of the opposite side of the mandible and parallel to the occlusal plane.

After positioning the needle the syringe is aspirated to check that there is no draw-back of blood from a punctured vessel before proceeding. If there is evidence of this the needle must be withdrawn slightly, the angle changed minimally and then advanced and tried again. Once all is well the agent is slowly injected, taking 30–45 sec, maintaining verbal contact and control. Unlike the case of the adult, the inferior dental block in children often gives buccal anaesthesia too, otherwise it is necessary to give a buccal infiltration to ensure anaesthesia of the long buccal nerve for dental extractions or other procedures which involve the buccal mucosa.

4. Intraligamentous

Instant anaesthesia is obtained when 0.2 ml doses of solution are injected directly down into the tooth's periodontal ligament, mesially and distally, via a 30 gauge needle using a special pressure syringe, e.g. Citoject (Bayer) or Ligmaject (Figure 5.3). The injection will not cause lip anaesthesia and there is no danger of intravascular injection. The syringe shape allows the bulk of the syringe to be concealed in the hand. Thus the technique presents several advantages for use in children.

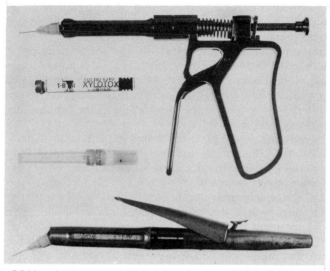

Figure 5.3 Ligmaject (*upper*) and Citoject (*lower*) syringes for intraligamentous injections

However, any infection of the gingival sulcus may be driven deeper into the periodontal structures and result in a possible post-injection periodontal abscess. The volume of injected solution must be strictly limited for an excess can cause the tooth to become extruded slightly from the socket and may result in after-pain. It is suggested that the technique be reserved for cases with a healthy periodontium or as a supplemental anaesthetic method in resistant cases. Otherwise this technique can be considered for extraction cases.

After care

Always make sure that there will be no trauma to the anaesthetized tissues. Warn the child and the parent to protect the numb areas. It is a great temptation for a child to keep nibbling and squeezing the 'rubbery' lip. Also make it quite clear that the child must not eat or take very hot drinks, etc., until the anaesthetic has completely worn off (in about an hour after injection in most cases). All too often, a celebratory trip to the local hamburger restaurant on the way home from a dental appointment has resulted in injury to the anaesthetized parts when the child has bitten himself unawares. The operator should bear this postanaesthetic problem in mind at the time of injection and try to give the minimum amount of solution necessary for the operation in order to speed the recovery time.

Should such an injury occur there may be considerable swelling of the lip. The parent should be reassured that the condition will resolve quickly in a day or two. Meanwhile the abraded, bitten surface should be kept clean with chlorhexidine mouthwashes, and can be protected by regular application of carmellose sodium paste (Orobase ointment). Rarely does the self-inflicted wound of this sort require antibiotic therapy.

Sedation

Simple dental sedation is defined by the Expert Working Party on General Anaesthesia, Sedation and Resuscitation in Dentistry (the Poswillo report) as follows:

'A carefully controlled technique in which a single intravenous drug, or a combination of oxygen and nitrous oxide, is used to reinforce hypnotic suggestion and reassurance in a way which allows dental treatment to be performed with minimal physiological and psychological stress, but which allows verbal contact with the patient to be maintained at all times. The technique must carry a margin of safety wide enough to render unintended loss of consciousness unlikely'.

● Any technique of sedation other than as defined above must be regarded as coming within the meaning of dental general anaestheisa.

Oral sedation (see Chapter 15)

Anxiolytics are minor tranquillizers; sedatives relieve anxiety but produce lethargy and drowsiness; hypnotics promote sleep. There seems to be no clear boundary between these descriptive titles for in many cases their effect is dose-related.

Most of them are to be taken orally and, if prescribed as a single dose, their effect can be unpredictable in the young. Their action is affected by the dose, the rate of absorption, the rate of elimination by the liver, the constituents of the last meal and by the extent of the child's apprehension and fear. The nervous child's tense gastro-intestinal tract tends to absorb the drug slowly and it may thus be ineffective when needed at the time of the dental appointment. If the absorbed amount is inadequate it tends to remove the final restraint from the child and render it totally untreatable, or if excessive it will render the child unconscious.

Perhaps the best regime, where appropriate, is to give one dose of the drug (e.g. diazepam) at bedtime on the previous evening followed by a second dose immediately after breakfast and a third an hour before the dental appointment. The child then gets an unworried, good night's sleep and the relaxed gut allows normal drug absorption next morning so that the child is rendered sedate and docile in the surgery.

However, the after-effects and hangover from even a single dose of most of these drugs may last for many hours before they are cleared from the body and multiple doses can accumulate in the tissues. This slow recovery will affect the child's ability to look after himself on public roads etc. or to return to school. The child *must* be accompanied and kept under observation during this period. Drugs to relieve acute dental anxiety should only be given once or at the most intermittently, never as a regular thing, because they can cause dependence.

There is a wide range of suitable drugs available and the prescriber's choice will obviously be affected by his own personal experience and preference. Currently the most popular drugs are the chloral hydrate derivatives or the benzodiazepines. It is inadvisable to administer mixtures of any of these drugs.

Intravenous sedation

This is not recommended for children because of unpredictable reactions to the drugs, together with the practical difficulties of lack of cooperation and small veins. Relative analgesia is safer and easier to administer.

Relative analgesia (RA)

Conscious sedation using a gas and air, gas and oxygen inhalation method has been available for some two decades. A special apparatus has been developed for use in the dental surgery which can control the mixture of nitrous oxide and oxygen in such a way that there is never any danger of the concentration of oxygen falling below 30% and thus there is no possibility of the patient losing consciousness completely. The gases can be rapidly cleared from the patient's system and thus the technique has a high safety factor. This means that it can be administered by the operator himself.

There is a minimum requirement that a second appropriate person is present throughout, such as an experienced, trained dental surgery assistant capable of monitoring the patient's clinical condition and assisting the dentist in case of emergency. In addition, adequate facilities for the resuscitation of the patient must be available and both the dentist and his staff trained in their use.

Advantages
Relative analgesia is a safe, rapidly reversible technique useful for both children and adults.

Patients can resume normal activities 30 min after recovery, although it is advisable for a child to be escorted home.

Benefits
Relative analgesia can be used to relax the anxious, fearful patient and dull the sensation of dental treatment. In addition it causes partial amnesia, a raised pain threshold and a loss of the sense of the passage of time.

The operator gains from the depression of the patient's gag reflex and relaxation of tight oral musculature.

The patient returns more readily for future treatment.

Contraindications
Relative analgesia does not reduce the oxygen intake to a low limit and so contraindications are few.

The patient must be old enough to understand the benefits of the procedure and willing to cooperate.

Relative analgesia should *not* be used in cases of:

Multiple sclerosis or myasthenia gravis
Upper respiratory infections,
    even a 'cold'
    blocked nasal airway
       e.g. enlarged adenoids and tonsils
Complicated cardiac disease
Pulmonary disease
    e.g. emphysema, bronchiectasis
Pregnancy
Complicated drug therapy
Active psychiatric treatment.

Technique synopsis
Caution—Operators intending to use relative analgesia should: (a) Read the recommendations of the Poswillo report (1990), (b) Read Langa (1976) and Roberts (1990), (c) Experience inhalation sedation for themselves, and (d) Conduct at least their first 10 cases under the supervision of an experienced colleague.

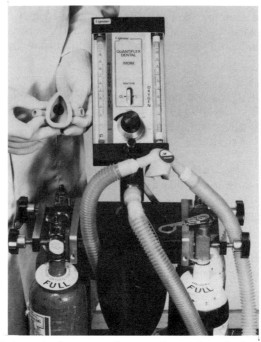

Figure 5.4 Relative analgesia apparatus incorporating passive antipollution tubing attached to the nosepiece. A second nosepiece is displayed on the left

Apparatus

Administration of inhalation sedation requires apparatus with incorporated fail-safe devices such as the Ohmeda Quantiflex Dental Monitored Dial Mixer (MDM) Relative Analgesia apparatus (Figure 5.4) which will not allow nitrous oxide to flow unless there is a simultaneous delivery of oxygen at the preset level of 3 litres/minute. Should the oxygen fail then the nitrous oxide is immediately cut off. An antipollution system should be used to scavange the waste gases from the surgery atmosphere (Ohmeda, UK Distributor, Nesor Products, Claremont Hall, Pentonville Place, London, N1).

Check the apparatus before the patient arrives. Check the dials and that the oxygen cut out is working. Make sure that the 'in use' gas cylinders are turned on and that there are full cylinders attached and available with a cylinder key.

Always have another adult present throughout, who is fully trained in resuscitation methods. Make sure that the resuscitation equipment is immediately to hand within arm's reach of the operator.

Preparation

Check the medical history.

First explain the procedure to the child and to the parent. Offer it to them and then allow the parent to persuade you to try it.

Informed consent to treatment under dental sedation must be obtained in writing on every occasion. A parent or responsible guardian must sign for minors under the age of 16.

Although relative analgesia may be given after a light meal it is best to keep the patient's food intake down during the four hours before this treatment.

The child should be accompanied by an adult.

Administration

Be reassuring and encouraging. Explain again what is about to happen. Demonstrate the nosepiece while it is disconnected from the apparatus (nosepieces come in several different sizes; choose one that is appropriate).

Get the patient comfortably positioned in the supine position, fingers intertwined. Switch on the pure oxygen and adjust the flow to slow speed, say 4–5 litres/minute. Lower the nosepiece over the patient's nose as you will have previously shown in the explanation and adjust it to fit comfortably. In most cases the patient can help here.

Adjust the gas flow control until the rebreathing bag is moving easily in time with the respiration. If the bag is deflated all the time the flow rate should be increased. If the bag is ballooning fully all the time then the rate of flow has to be reduced. This adjustment has to be made for each individual patient. The leakage of gases via oral breathing, talking, etc. will vary a lot.

After a minute or so, with the patient relaxed, and the nosepiece in place, it can be held there by sliding up the double tube clamp behind the headrest. Now the gas mixture is adjusted. Slowly titrate the nitrous oxide into the oxygen: 15% nitrous oxide for 1 minute, then 25% nitrous oxide for 1 minute, then 30% for 1 minute, thus administering increments of 5% per minute. The continuous flow system balances the total flow rate of the changing mixture of gases to that already selected. Gradually increase the nitrous oxide level, all the time talking quietly to the patient and monitoring his responses. The reduction in oxygen tension means that the patient will begin to experience a warm, tingling sensation in the peripheral circulation of the fingers and toes which gradually extends centrally.

Tell the patient to imagine that he is relaxing on a sunny beach and gradually feeling warm and relaxed and tingling. Establish verbal responses from the patient: 'Can you feel the tingle in your toes and feet?—Good—And in your fingers, too?' 'Can you feel it moving slowly up your legs to your tummy and chest?–Good', and so on. This sensation takes a few minutes to occur with the operator slowly titrating and balancing the gas mixture and flow as required.

Finally, the patient reaches a stage where they begin to feel slightly disorientated, 'floating' and lethargic and it seems to be a great effort to respond to your questions. Yet they are still able to respond, albeit slowly and can cooperate by moving slowly and opening their mouth if requested to. The cough reflex remains unimpaired, so to that extent the airway is protected.

Assess the depth of the sedation from the patient's appearance and by their experience of the 'tingling all over' and/or floating sensation. Having reached this state, the child's cooperation is assured. However, despite some degree of analgesia and post-operative amnesia, dental treatment of a painful nature, e.g. deep cavity preparations, extractions etc. still require the administration of a local anaesthetic injection, but now even the most nervous child will not be bothered to refuse the injection or require persuasion to accept it.

Although the safety of the apparatus design means that it may be used by the operator without the presence of an anaesthetist, it is important that a check is made from time to time on the patient's responses. The open mouth can allow the gases to escape at an uncontrolled rate and this will affect the level of analgesia obtained. Thus the operator has to be alert and ready to change the gas setting from time to time.

As the end of the session arrives, it is usual to begin to reduce the nitrous oxide level gradually so that the patient has almost completely recovered as the work in the mouth is completed. Finally allow the patient to breathe 100% oxygen for 2 minutes. The child is allowed to lie in the chair, supine, for a few minutes and then sit up gradually. Ask them to sit in a recovery room for ten minutes and check them again personally before discharging them. Record the nitrous oxide level required for future reference.

After-effects from relative analgesia are few. Occasionally a patient complains of a slight headache for a few minutes but this is a rare and transient occurrence.

Relative analgesia provides a valuable method of helping patients to overcome great dental fear and anxiety, in order to carry out urgent treatment and to get the mouth into a reasonable condition quickly. However, in most cases, once such preliminary stages of treatment have been carried out, this method ought not to become the expected norm for every treatment session.

General anaesthesia

The use of full general anaesthesia for the dental treatment of children has decreased in recent years as the need for multiple extractions has been reduced. It should be avoided wherever possible.

The General Dental Council in its Amendment to the Notice for the Guidance of Dentists, May 1989, and now the Poswillo report set out clear conditions with regard to the use of general anaesthesia in dental practice. These direct that only a dental or medical practitioner appropriately trained and experienced in the use of anaesthetic drugs for dental purposes may administer a general anaesthetic for dental treatment. That person must be other than the dentist carrying out the treatment and he must remain with the patient throughout the whole anaesthetic procedure and until the patient's protective reflexes have returned. Neither general anaesthesia nor sedation should be employed unless proper equipment for their administration is used and adequate facilities for the resuscitation of the patient, including basic life support equipment, are readily available with both dentist and staff fully trained and rehearsed in their use.

General anaesthetics for children's dental treatment should be restricted to specialist practices and hospital departments where the operating conditions can fulfil these necessary obligations and where experienced staff, full back-up, patient monitoring apparatus and emergency resuscitation equipment are immediately available.

Referral for general anaesthesia

The technique is used in cases where the patient cannot be expected to cooperate, e.g. for very young children; for the mentally or emotionally handicapped; for multiple extractions in various quadrants of the mouth; where there is doubt about obtaining adequate local analgesia; and where there is severe infection.

In addition to the usual referral letter, relevant radiographs and appointment arrangements, the referring dentist must check the patient's medical history carefully to make sure that there is no contraindication to general anaesthesia and if in doubt should discuss the matter with the child's doctor and the anaesthetist before proceeding further.

Consent

Informed consent to general anaesthesia must be given in writing and signed by the parent or responsible guardian on every occasion for minors under the age of 16 years. This is usually obtained on a standard form.

Pre-operation

The child must not have had anything to eat or drink for a prolonged period (at least six hours) before the administration of the anaesthetic. This is to ensure that possible vomiting while the patient is unconscious does not threaten the airway.

On arrival at the surgery the patient must be accompanied by an adult who will be responsible for ensuring that the child is accompanied home again after the operation.

Day-stay

A day-stay outpatient may be given endotracheal intubation anaesthesia for an early morning operation and after recovery be allowed to go home on that same afternoon. This type of anaesthetic should only be given when there is the back-up possibility of admission to a hospital ward if the need arises and the patient is not fit to be discharged within the prescribed time. It should only be undertaken in specialist hospital departments.

Intubation on a day-stay basis is *not* considered to be suitable for small children, for they have a small trachea and in the event of any postoperative laryngeal oedema they would rapidly develop respiratory distress and be in a life-threatening state. This may occur at any time during the following 24 hours or so and thus a child needs to be admitted to hospital for it has to remain under special supervision for this long postanaesthetic period.

Day-stay intubation anaesthesia is used for operations lasting obout one hour, e.g. for full mouth rehabilitation, the extraction of unerupted teeth, treatment of cysts, root canal therapy and apicectomy, etc.

Chapter 6

Restorative dentistry

Dry field

The ability to obtain a dry operating field is essential for many aspects of restorative dental treatment:

1. For clear vision.
2. For asepsis.
3. To allow materials (e.g. cements, sealants, restorative materials) to set properly without moisture contamination.

Methods

1. Cotton wool rolls: These are available in various diameters and can be cut into appropriate lengths and shapes. Their retention may be improved by the use of cotton wool roll clamps (e.g. those made by Pulpadent).
2. Virilium dry guards and Scandent dry tips: Both have the advantage of being thin and thus they occupy less space in the sulcus. They are available in small and large sizes.
3. Saliva ejectors: For children these should be small, light and smooth and, if possible, soft. An ejector with a lingual flange is useful to keep the tongue away from an adjacent mandibular tooth.
4. High velocity, low vacuum central suction tubes can evacuate air-rotor aerosols and water sprays efficiently. However, the child needs to be gradually introduced to the sound and the cooling air current of the 'dentist's vacuum cleaner' to avoid causing unnecessary fear.
5. Rubber dam, the best of all. It is probably not used enough because of inexperience in the operators, although this can only be overcome by practice!

Rubber dam

Contraindications

A very uncooperative, nervous or inexperienced child.
Some medical or physical conditions, e.g. asthma.
Severe gingival inflammation.

Advantages

Controls movements of the tongue and cheek.
Protects the airway and prevents items being inhaled.
Protects the tissues from trauma, chemicals and tastes.
Keeps out sprays and high-velocity suckers.
Improves vision of the operating site.
Improves standards of operating and restoration.
Stops contamination of pulp treatment and restorative materials.
Reduces delays in rinsing out, etc.

Equipment (Figure 6.1)

1. Rubber dam. Heavy duty (less likely to tear), dark colour: such as black and green (shows up well the teeth and tissues by contrast). Some dams are flavoured.
2. Rubber dam punch.
3. Rubber dam clamp forceps.
4. Rubber dam clamps.
   The precise choice of clamps will vary with different operators who will develop their own preferences, e.g. a basic set of clamps might include:

Permanent molars	ASH	AW	BW	K	(W = Wingless)
Primary molars	ASH	FW	HW	G	
Incisors and canines	ASH	EW	C	E	

   Wingless clamps have an advantage in applying the dam, but wings tend to hold the rubber down for a better view of the tooth.
5. Waxed dental floss to tie clamp and the dam.
6. A lightweight rubber dam frame (such as Ash or Young's RD frame).
7. A method of marking where to punch the holes (a stamp or a pencil).
8. A pleasant tasting lubricating cream such as brushless shaving cream or petroleum jelly may be used to ease the dam between

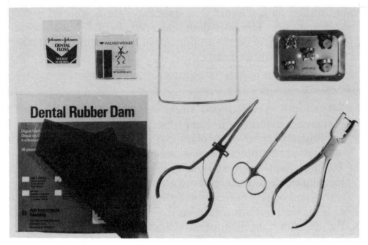

Figure 6.1 Some of the items needed to apply the rubber dam

tight, dry contact points more readily. However, this is rarely needed for the teeth are already moist with saliva.

9. Dental napkin to pad under the dam.
10. Blunt-nosed scissors.
11. Wooden wedges/tooth picks/strips of rubber dam 3 mm wide to wedge the dam down into place between erupted teeth.
12. A flat plastic instrument.
13. A small rubber mouth prop.

Preparation

It is necessary to anaesthetize the area first. Local anaesthesia is probably required for the cavity restoration and in case pulp therapy is needed, but it is also needed to reduce the possible pain of pressure of the clamp and dam near the gingival margin.

Tell the child what will happen. Adapt the explanation to the age of the child. Use terms like 'button', 'raincoat', 'parcel' etc.

Method

Mark the positions of the teeth to be isolated on the rubber, locating them so that the teeth will be near the centre of the dam.

To facilitate application by the inexperienced operator the holes for two adjacent teeth can be punched so that they overlap, or instead, two adjacent holes may be joined by cutting the intervening strand of dam with scissors. The dam can then be slipped over the clamp very easily. The final dam may seep slightly, but the ease of application can increase the confidence of both operator and patient for future use of rubber dam.

Method A

1. Select tooth to be clamped. In the buccal quadrant either the 1st permanent molar or the 2nd primary molar is preferable, for the 1st primary molar or primary canine are not ideal. Choose an appropriate clamp: a wingless one preferably.
2. Tie the clamp with at least a 12 inch length of dental floss looping the floss through both clamp holes (this means that the clamp can be prevented from falling into the throat if it slips off or if the clamp fractures across the bow). (Figure 6.2.)
3. Put the clamp on the tooth and adjust it to the correct position. Remove clamp forceps.
4. Stretch the lubricated rubber dam with fingers and thumb and pass it over the attached clamp. This is easier if a wingless clamp has been used. When safely in position carry the prepared holes over the other selected teeth and place a wedge or rubber strip in the appropriate contact area between two teeth to hold the dam in position (Figure 6.3b). Alternatively, secure the dam with floss, using a double surgeon's loop pulled tight by an assistant as you work it down into position with a flat plastic instrument, and then secured with a further knot.
5. Pull the floss attached to the clamp from below the dam to the operator's side. Then if the clamp has to be removed later, e.g. to place a matrix band, the dam will not be displaced by the

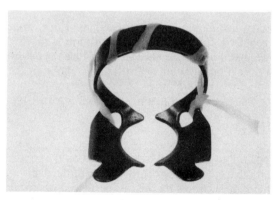

Figure 6.2 Rubber dam clamp with dental floss attached prior to positioning it in the mouth

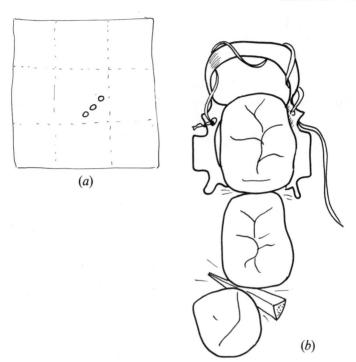

Figure 6.3 (*a*) Punch the holes near the centre of the rubber dam; (*b*) A wooden wedge may be used to hold the rubber dam in position

floss at that stage.
6. Attach a light dam frame to hold the rubber away from the face.
7. Place a dental napkin under the dam against the skin.
8. Check if a saliva ejector will be needed. Most children can manage to swallow with the dam in position.
9. Check that the patient can breathe easily.
10. If the patient is biting hard on the clamp use a small rubber mouth prop on the other side 'to lean on' or as 'an armchair for the teeth'.

Method B
This is for the more experienced operator.

1. Prior to application a winged clamp, prepared with dental floss as before, is positioned in the appropriate hole punched in the rubber dam.

2. The dam frame is also attached to the rubber.
3. The whole assembly is applied to the tooth.
4. With the clamp in position, the dam is flicked off its wings with a flat plastic instrument and the operator positions the rest of the dam in the usual manner.

Where the preparation for a Class II restoration means extending towards the gingival margin interproximally and possibly impinging on the rubber dam (a) cut the rubber and allow for the slight seepage, or (b) wedge the space with a wooden wedge that the bur can work against.

When a Class II preparation is to be restored in a tooth already clamped the clamp can get in the way of the matrix band. With care, the clamp can be removed (if you haven't pulled the floss through as suggested previously the dam will be displaced!) and the matrix positioned to replace the function of the clamp.

Removing the rubber dam means removing the wedges, cutting the retaining floss (not that on the clamp!), perhaps cutting the dam alongside new restorations and removing clamp and frame in one. Always check that all the dam has been removed and that none has been torn off and remains in the interdental space. Review the protected tissues again before dismissing the patient.

Restorative dentistry for primary teeth
Aims

Maintenance of arch length and healthy oral environment; prevention and relief of pain; maintenance and improvement of appearance (Kennedy, 1986).

General principles

Consider:

1. The patient
Age. Medical history. Previous prevention and treatment experience. Ability to accept treatment. Expected cooperation. Rapport with operator.

2. The mouth environment
Standard of oral hygiene. Caries experience. Access to the tooth.

3. The tooth
History. Appearance. Extent of caries.

Results of special tests: vitality test (not often of use in primary teeth as (a) the patient may not understand it and respond erratically, and

(b) normal root resorption brings degeneration of the pulp inner-
vation), transillumination, radiograph.

Anatomy of the tooth. The primary teeth differ from permanent
teeth anatomically, particularly with regard to pulp size, tooth size,
external contour and in their time span in the mouth. The primary
tooth has a large pulp with long pulp horns and is at risk with
high-speed instrumentation.

4. Treatment choice
Does the tooth really require operative treatment? Some minimal,
non-penetrating, surface lesions may be arrested by the effects of
suitable diet adjustment, improved oral hygiene and topical fluoride
treatment. Some cavities are hard and self-cleansing. Alternatively,
the tooth may be beyond restoration and require extraction.

5. Anaesthetic
An appropriate anaesthetic should be given before any anticipated
painful procedures, e.g. most cavity preparations, the application of
matrix bands and rubber dam clamps, etc. The resultant analgesia
eliminates the sensation of pain, but the noise and sensations of
pressure remain and the tissues need to be handled gently.

6. Dry field/vision
Isolate, dry and illuminate the tooth adequately during operative
treatment and to ensure adequate vision. Fibreoptic light via the
handpiece is now available.

7. Instrumentation
All instruments should be used with a light touch and with an
explanation of the noise to be anticipated by the patient. A child's
growing experience of cavity preparation is best developed in a
series of increasingly noisy steps: hand instruments, then on slow
engine instruments and finally to the use of the air-turbine.

8. Available restorative materials
Over recent decades these have changed in internal structure and
composition, and in working properties. New adhesive techniques
mean that cavity preparations may not need to be as extensive as
before in order to gain retention and strength, although amalgam
still demands that the cavity is made retentive and undercut. New
spherical amalgam alloys may be packed into rounded corners in
cavities and are strong enough not to require extensive cavity
preparations to provide bulk strength. The cavosurface angle is

important for amalgam, but this is not so with adhesive materials such as glass ionomer cement.

Cavity classification

Cavities in teeth are still conveniently described using the traditional Black's classification:

Class I	Cavities originating in anatomical pits, fissures and structural defects of premolar and molar teeth.
Class II	Cavities originating on the proximal surfaces of premolars and molars.
Class III	Cavities originating on the proximal surfaces of incisors, not involving the incisal angle, and canines.
Class IV	Cavities originating on the proximal surfaces of incisors involving the incisal angle.
Class V	Cavities originating on the gingival third of labial, palatal, buccal or lingual surfaces of the teeth.

(Note: Black was describing the surface of the tooth where the caries attacked, not the final cavity preparation. Nowadays his cavity designs are generally considered to be too extensive and destructive of sound tooth structure.)

Cavity preparation

(*Eye protection.* Any patient in the supine position in the dental chair should wear protective glasses to prevent accidental eye injury and to shield the eyes from bright operating lights.)

Class 1 (Pits, fissures and structural defects)

Access
Ideally, use a long head, plain cut, pear-shaped bur (Ash 21, US 331L) in a high-speed turbine to enter the cavity. This bur will penetrate enamel, remove caries and develop smooth, rounded undercuts that facilitate retention.

Establish depth
Initially, confine penetration to a depth of about 0.5 mm into the dentine.

Cavity outline
Begin to explore the outline of the extent of the caries. Keep the preparation as narrow as possible. Remember that extension of the cavity towards the cusps may endanger the pulp cornuae (Figure 6.4).

Retention
Consider which restorative material is to be used and plan an appropriate retentive shape. Develop the walls of the cavity keeping them convergent towards the occlusal surface to assist retention. Unless the tooth will soon be shed consider the judicious extension into adjacent fissures that are prone to further caries but remember that total 'extension for prevention' may be excessive and weaken the tooth.

Eliminate caries
Eliminate all remaining carious dentine using a round bur in a slow handpiece or sharp excavators. Check particularly along the walls and the amelodentinal junction. Keep all the internal angles rounded to avoid the pulp.

Finish margins
Remove all unsupported enamel. In all cavities to be restored with amalgam a cavosurface angle of 85–90° allows maximum marginal

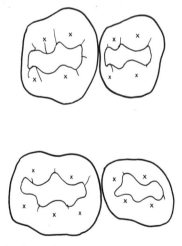

Figure 6.4 Class I occlusal cavity outlines in maxillary and mandibular molars. Cavities may not have to be as extensive as those illustrated (e.g. single pits) but will lie within these outlines. The cusps are indicated by 'X'; extending the cavity towards the cusps may endanger the pulp cornuae

strength to both amalgam and enamel and reduces the risk of early marginal failure of the restoration.

Class II (Proximal surfaces of premolars and molars)

This is perhaps the most important restoration of all. If it is badly contoured it may allow the adjacent teeth to drift; any cervical overhang will cause pain and gingivitis due to plaque retention. If the cavity is designed badly the restoration may be dislodged or fracture and slip from the cavity into the interdental space causing discomfort and damage to the interdental papilla.

1. This restoration usually requires a local anaesthetic, for preparation of the occlusal lock and matrix placement will be uncomfortable.
2. It is advisable to check the radiograph and estimate the depth of the caries and its proximity to the pulp. The cavity is generally more extensive than the area of radiolucency seen on the film.
3. For large cavities extending beyond two surfaces e.g. a mesio-occluso-distal with a lingual extension, or when a cusp has been lost, consider the use of a chrome-steel crown (see below).

Access
Gain access to the caries using the pear-shaped bur described for the Class I preparation.

Establish depth
Initially, confine penetration to a depth of about 0.5 mm into the dentine.

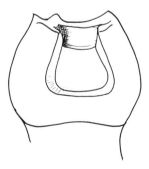

Figure 6.5 Class II cavity. Develop a curved cervical margin interproximally, below the contact point, but above the gingival level if possible

Cavity outline
Proceed to define the cavity outline and decide upon the restorative
material to be used. Amalgam is considered to be the best restorative material for the restoration of Class II cavities in primary
teeth.

1. Explore and remove the interproximal caries; trying to keep the
   opening of the embrasures to a minimum although extending
   them to self-cleansing areas; developing a curved cervical
   contour and if possible keeping this above the gingival contour
   (Figure 6.5), but below the contact point area. Deep extension
   cervically should be avoided if possible for the marked incurva-
   ture of the tooth will predispose pulpal exposure on the axial
   wall. Try to keep the walls of the cavity at right angles to
   the surface (Figure 6.6). Make sure the pulp is not cariously
   exposed; if it is, then the restoration will be combined with pulp
   therapy. The most likely point for an exposure of the pulp is
   again on the axial wall where the contour of the pulp chamber
   echoes the external contour of the tooth (Figure 6.7). In some
   cases slow caries may have stimulated the formation of secondary dentine and this will allow a deeper preparation to be made.
2. Next develop the occlusal lock. This may be prescribed by
   the extent of the caries, or it may need to be extended into
   non-carious enamel and dentine. The depth of the lock
   should not exceed 0.5 mm into the dentine in non-carious areas
   (Figure 6.8). The lock walls should be convergent towards the
   occlusal surface to aid retention, with rounded internal angles.
   This section must be extensive enough to support the interproximal section of the restoration and the whole strong
   enough at the isthmus between the occlusal and interproximal
   sections to resist fracture at this vulnerable point. Strength may
   come from either the width of the lock and isthmus or their
   depth, although the latter is limited by the size of the pulp. The
   isthmus may be half the width between the cusps; too wide and
   it will weaken the tooth, too narrow and the restoration may
   fracture at this point. The pulpal–axial line angle should be
   rounded.

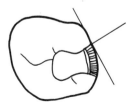

Figure 6.6 Class II cavity. Minimal
extension is made into self-cleansing
areas and the embrasure walls should
be finished at right angles to the
enamel surface

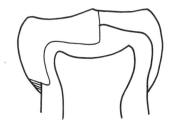

Figure 6.7 Class II cavity. Remember the direction of the enamel prisms when finishing the cervical margin. Keep the axial wall curved away from the pulp where it echoes the external tooth contour and round the pulpal-axial line angle to increase the strength of the restoration at this point

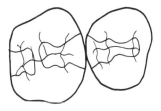

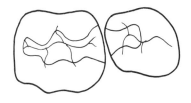

Figure 6.8 Class II cavity outlines in maxillary and mandibular molars

Retention
Retention will have been developed, but further retention for the interproximal box can be achieved by carefully developing shallow grooves, with a fine fissure bur, along the bucco-axial and linguo-axial line angles.

Eliminate caries
Eliminate all remaining carious dentine using a round bur in a slow handpiece or sharp excavators. Check along the walls and the amelodentinal junction paying particular attention to the embrasure walls. Keep all the internal angles rounded to avoid the pulp.

Finish margins
Finish the walls to remove all unsupported enamel and to develop appropriate cavosurface angle for the material chosen.

(The 'Tunnel Preparation' has been suggested. To preserve the marginal ridge in selected cases, the interproximal caries is approached and eliminated via a tunnel extending from the occlusal surface to reach the lesion. This method has been criticized because it is inappropriate for small primary teeth, does not allow clear visibility of the cavity margins, threatens exposure of the pulp and predisposes fracture of the marginal ridge.)

Class III (Proximal surfaces of incisors and canines)

Access
Enter the lesion with a small round or fissure bur in a slow handpiece. Where the teeth are spaced access is direct; where there is a tight contact point open the cavity by developing a lock in the thick middle third of the tooth. This lock is generally prepared on the palatal surface of the upper incisor and, partially for ease of access, on the labial of the lower incisor for, in addition, the pulp lies slightly further away from these surfaces.

Cavity outline
Proceed to define the extent of the caries (Figure 6.9). Take special care not to weaken the incisal edge of the tooth and to avoid pulp exposure.

Retention
This is dictated by the restorative material chosen. Where access to the cavity was made by developing a lock this will improve the retention of the larger restoration. The general inclination of the lock should be angled to take advantage of the direction of the primary enamel prisms (Figure 6.10).

Eliminate caries
Eliminate all remaining carious dentine using a round bur in a slow handpiece or sharp excavators. Check particularly along the walls and the amelodentinal junction. Keep all the internal angles rounded to avoid the pulp.

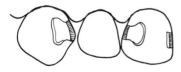

Figure 6.9 Class III cavity outlines in primary maxillary incisors and canine

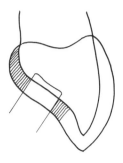

Figure 6.10 The walls of the retention lock should be finished at right angles to the tooth surface. Note the direction of the enamel prisms in this region

Finish margins
Be sparing in removal of enamel where an adhesive restorative material has been chosen otherwise remove all unsupported enamel and develop appropriate cavosurface angles.

Class IV (Proximal surfaces of incisors, involving the incisal angle)

A cavity of this size may indicate that pulpal involvement has already occurred. Check radiographs to ensure that there is no apical pathology that may put the permanent successor at risk.

Treatment choice
This will be affected by the extent of the lesion and the expected longevity of the tooth before exfoliation. Current thought tends towards the use of a strip crown in most cases, but the operator may sometimes find the Class IV restoration appropriate.

Access
Enter the lesion cautiously with a round bur in a slow handpiece.

Cavity outline
Proceed to define the cavity outline. Take care to avoid pulp exposure.

Retention
Although adhesive restorative materials are generally recommended, retention usually requires the development of a lock which, as in the Class III preparation is best placed on the palatal of the upper incisor and the labial of the lower. Keep the lock in the middle third of the cervical region if possible, where the tooth is thickest. In some cases retention requires the use of a pin which must be placed very carefully in the cervical margin to avoid pulpal

exposure. Where the retention is still questionable, a strip crown preparation may be more appropriate.

Eliminate caries
Eliminate all remaining carious dentine using a round bur in a slow handpiece or sharp excavators. Check particularly along the walls and the amelodentinal junction. Keep all the internal angles rounded to avoid the pulp.

Finish margins
As with the Class III preparation be sparing in removal of enamel where an adhesive restorative material has been chosen.

Class V (Gingival third of the labial, palatal, buccal or lingual surfaces of the teeth)

Many of these cavities can be found to be surprisingly deep and extensive and the operator should be alert to discover and treat them at an early stage if possible. Cavities on the labial surface of the maxillary incisors are easily accessible and simply restored and thus can be a good way of introducing a child to the procedures of restorative treatment.

Access
Enter the lesion cautiously with a round bur in a slow handpiece.

Establish depth
Initially, confine penetration to a depth of about 0.5 mm into the dentine.

Cavity outline
Proceed to define the extent of the cavity outline. This is usually accomplished with a flat fissure bur held at right angles to the tooth surface, sometimes with a small inverted cone bur. The cervical wall of the cavity usually follows the gingival contour. Where the caries extends subgingivally in a partially erupted tooth the cavity may have to be filled temporarily until the tooth is fully erupted.

Retention
This is again dictated by the restorative material chosen, but amalgam will require an undercut cavity. Retentive undercuts should be confined to the cervical and occlusal walls only.

Eliminate caries
Eliminate all remaining carious dentine using a round bur in a slow handpiece or sharp excavators. Check particularly along the walls and the amelodentinal junction. Keep all the internal angles rounded to avoid the pulp.

Finish margins
Finish the walls to remove all unsupported enamel and to develop appropriate cavosurface angle for the material chosen. The cervical margin may be finished with a narrow chisel where the cavity extends below the gingival margin.

(*'Discing'* and *'Saucerisation'*. In certain rare cases, where a tooth is soon to be exfoliated, shallow caries may be treated by discing, grinding and modifying the shape of the tooth to render it self-cleansing, applying topical fluoride to the surface, e.g. Duraphat varnish, and monitoring the tooth until it is shed. The aesthetic appearance of teeth treated in this way is usually very poor.)

Cavity lining

Protect the pulp against thermal or chemical irritation with a thin layer of a quick-setting calcium hydroxide base (e.g. Dycal: Amalgamated Dental Co.). In many cases there is little room to place a cement lining in a primary tooth without sacrificing the bulk and strength of the permanent restoration.

Matrices

Class II

When packing this restoration it is most important to ensure proper gingival contouring and a matrix is mandatory. Narrow Siqveland or Tofflemire matrices, or less bulky T-bands may be chosen. Some operators prefer custom-made spot-welded strip bands. In every case wedging of the cervical margin must be considered to avoid the packed amalgam slipping through a loosely adapted band.

Class III

Celluloid matrices, wedged cervically and held firmly into place with the fingers are used for resin and glass-ionomer restorations. Being transparent they allow the operator to ensure the adequate packing of material and also facilitate light curing. Distal cavities in canines are generally filled with amalgam in which case a metal matrix strip is required to resist the packing pressure involved.

Class IV

Again wedged celluloid matrices may be used, although they cannot control all the surfaces completely and the resulting restoration will require careful contouring and finishing. A strip crown may be considered in these cases.

Choices of restorative material

Amalgam is still the material most commonly used for Class I and Class II, distal Class III cavities in canines, and for some Class V cavities where it is not aesthetically contraindicated. The properties of new alloys give increased strength and resistance to marginal breakdown. Amalgam, being radio-opaque, is easily differentiated from recurrent caries in any subsequent radiographs.

Composite resins may be used to restore all classes of cavity, but apart from their good aesthetic appearance they do not have superior physical properties to amalgam and are less wear resistant. The acid-etch technique is used and it must be remembered that primary enamel has to be etched for twice the time recommended for etching permanent enamel.

Glass-ionomer cements (GIC). These are hybrid composite materials composed of ion-leachable glass powder dispersed in a cross-linked polyacrylate matrix. The manufacturers suggest that these materials may be used to restore all classes of cavity in primary teeth. After the cavity walls have been cleared of microscopic debris with an acid conditioner the material has adhesive properties to both dentine and enamel, which gives it a good marginal seal, and also allows it to be considered for otherwise non-retentive cavities. In addition glass-ionomer cements leach fluoride to the cavity margins and adjacent teeth. They have a reasonable aesthetic appearance. However, these materials are very technique-demanding, and very few reports on controlled clinical studies of their use in Class II cavities have been published.

Completion of restoration

Contour
Contour the restorative material and allow it to set properly.

Check

Remove matrix and the isolating materials or rubber dam, check the margins and occlusion and make any necessary adjustments.

Protect

Warn the child and parent to allow an amalgam to set for at least an hour before eating on it.

Finish

Composites and glass-ionomer cements may be finished at the same visit with white stones and flexible discs coated with petroleum jelly. Do not use a water spray for a GIC restoration and coat it with varnish again afterwards. Recall the child in due course (after at least two days) to polish amalgam restoration.

Monitor

Review the condition of the restoration at subsequent visits.

Preformed crowns for primary teeth

Stainless-steel crowns

Indications

1.   Rampant caries involving more than three surfaces of the tooth.
2.   Primary tooth after pulp therapy may have weakened it.
3.   Hypoplastic enamel, dentinogenesis imperfecta, etc.
4.   Abutment for a space maintainer.

Choice

In general, the available size selection, precision and finish have improved. They are not often used for anterior teeth because of the poor aesthetic appearance, and strip crowns have superseded them here.

Two kinds of steel crowns are available. One is untrimmed and allows the operator scope to festoon the cervical margin and to stretch and contour the overall shape to his own requirements. The second kind are 'pre-finished' molar crowns (e.g. ion Ni-Chro; 3M) (Figure 6.11) with a constricted cervix, and are pre-trimmed, pre-crimped and pre-belled to give a good anatomical contour. They have been work-hardened during manufacture and given a feathered cervical edge. They should only need minor adjustment to tighten the fit and are thus much quicker to apply.

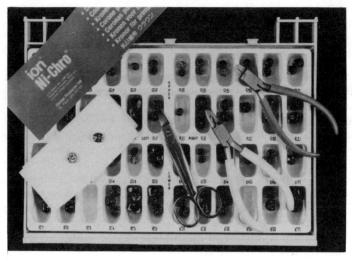

Figure 6.11 A selection of ion Ni-Chro crowns for primary teeth

Preparation

Tooth

1. Remove caries.
2. Place a sub-base of calcium hydroxide.
3. Restore the tooth with reinforced zinc oxide/eugenol or a phosphate cement.
4. Clear the interproximal spaces with a tapered fissure bur or stone, taking care not to develop an interproximal shoulder or abrade the adjacent tooth. If the preparation is being done under a rubber dam, place a wooden wedge in the interdental space to avoid cutting the dam.
5. Make a minimal reduction of the buccal and lingual walls; just to the gingival contour.
6. Reduce the occlusal surface by 1–1.5 mm.
7. Smooth all sharp edges.
8. The final shape to aim for is a 'smaller tooth', but make sure that no cervical shoulders or ledges remain and that the occlusal reduction follows the normal contours of the tooth.

Crown   Crown selection. Measure the space accurately with callipers and select a crown that will fit neatly over the prepared tooth and re-establish proper mesiodistal relationship.

Where necessary trim and adjust the crown margins with scissors or crown shears and pliers (a special range is available), taking care to protect the patient's eyes from flying fragments of metal. Polish the crown margins again.

Fitting. Use light to moderate finger pressure to seat the crown to obtain a 'snap' fit. If this moderate pressure will not seat a pre-finished crown, select one a size larger, for a crown that has been forced into place under excessive pressure will be very difficult to remove. If a selected pre-formed crown is too long, but the cervical opening is correct, select one size smaller and trim and crimp it to obtain the desired fit. The properly contoured crown will snap into position with its edges 1 mm below the gingival margin and cause no pressure blanching of the gingiva. The occlusion should be checked and in some cases it may be necessary to remove more of the occlusal surface of the tooth to allow the crown to be seated at the appropriate level. This adjustment can be facilitated by using indicating paste in the crown.

Cementation

Remove the crown from the tooth, wash and dry it, and polish any burred edges that could act as plaque traps. Clean, dry and isolate the tooth. Apply a thin mix of high strength, small particle cement (such as crown and bridge cement) to the inside of the crown and to the tooth. Too thick a mix of cement cannot flow past a well con-toured crown margin and this will prevent the crown from seating properly. Insert the crown and get the child to press it firmly in place by biting carefully on a cotton wool roll or a wooden tongue depressor. Then quickly check the occlusion and if all is well continue the gentle biting pressure until the cement has set. Check the margins and remove excess cement, flossing between the teeth (perhaps with a knot in the floss) to ensure that none remains interdentally.

Cautions

Some authorities advise the use of a rubber dam when inserting steel crowns to avoid the danger of ingestion or inhalation if they are lost in the mouth.

If a steel crown is improperly contoured at the cervical margin it will cause gingival inflammation and tissue degeneration due to plaque retention.

Steel crowns should not be considered to be long-term resto-rations for permanent teeth for they tend to cause periodontal problems. Cast crowns are preferred for children over the age of 15 years.

Strip crowns (e.g. Unitek Pedoform crown forms; 3M Health Care, 3M House, Morley Street, Loughborough, Leicestershire LE11 1EP. (0509 611611))

These transparent crown forms simplify composite work for paedodontic anterior restoration. Trimmed and filled with either chemical or light-curing restorative material they contour the material and support it while it sets and then strip off easily leaving a smooth surface.

Preparation

Tooth

1. Clean tooth with non-fluoridated prophylaxis paste.
2. Check the shade of the restoration required.
3. Reduce tooth surfaces, incisal length and interproximally to allow crown form to fit over tooth. Consider preparing a circumferential retention groove in the cervical third.
4. Remove remaining caries.
5. Maintain a dry field.
6. Protect pulp with appropriate material.

Crown

1. Select appropriate crown and trim margins with scissors.
2. Try the crown over the tooth to check contour and margins.
3. Make a small hole vent in the palatal side.

Etching

1. Etch the enamel for the appropriate time with etching solution or gel. Note: The enamel of primary teeth takes longer to etch than that of permanent teeth.
2. Wash the tooth for 30 sec with the water syringe, then dry it with the air syringe and check that the enamel has become chalky white indicating a proper etch.

Positioning

1. Apply an appropriate adhesive to the tooth.
2. Fill the crown form with restorative material, avoiding or venting any air bubbles.
3. Place the filled crown on the prepared tooth, pressing it into position with the fingers.
4. Quickly remove any excess material with a probe, checking the interproximal areas particularly.

5.   Allow the material to cure and set or commence the light curing cycle (the crowns are transparent).

Removal
When the material has hardened, cut through the crown form with a probe or fine scaler, starting at the cervical margin, and strip it off, leaving a matrix-smooth surface.

Finishing
Check the cervical margins and the occlusion carefully and make any necessary adjustments before dismissing the patient.

Endodontic treatment for primary teeth

It is important to try to avoid premature extraction of pulpally involved primary teeth, to allow the child 'to eat, speak, smile and grow' with them. In particular, the premature loss of molar teeth will not only limit the child's diet choices, but it will also tend to exaggerate any crowding tendencies, whereas a successfully pulp-treated tooth is a perfect space maintainer.

The anatomy of the tooth presents special difficulties in the endodontic treatment of the primary molar teeth. The thin flattened roots have erratic pulp canals with branching and connecting fibrils and apical ramifications which makes complete mechanical removal of all pulp tissue impossible. In addition, the curved molar root presents mechanical problems and the danger of perforation in instrumentation by all but the most flexible broaches and files. During normal root resorption prior to exfoliation the apical opening begins to lie more coronally on the bifurcation aspect than the apparent apex of the root. It must be remembered during all considerations of treatment for the primary tooth that the developing permanent tooth germ lies in close proximity and will be affected adversely by associated infection, aggressive instrumentation, leaking medicaments or non-resorbable materials.

(Practice endodontic techniques on extracted teeth first to reacquaint yourself with the anatomy and 'feel' of the root canals. Examine the tooth's internal structure with a magnifying glass. Section the teeth as well.)

General considerations

Parent
Ensure that the parent is fully informed about the proposed treatment, is motivated towards saving the tooth and will reliably

keep the necessary appointments to complete and monitor the procedure. Unfortunately, some parents still opt for extraction.

Child

1. General Health. Pulp therapy may be contraindicated in certain cases, e.g. cardiac abnormality, kidney disease, etc. Alternatively, it may be strongly indicated where there is a need to avoid extractions or general anaesthesia, e.g. blood dyscrasias, respiratory problems, etc.
2. Cooperation. This kind of treatment takes time, generally requires local anaesthesia and, preferably, the application of rubber dam. Can this child be expected to react well and accept these procedures?
3. General Dental Condition. Does the condition of the mouth contraindicate pulp therapy, e.g. the presence of grossly neglected teeth and multiple carious exposures or abscesses? Is the tooth due to be shed normally anyway?

Pulpal diagnosis

History

Pain   Sometimes pulpal pathology remains subclinical, there is no history of pain, and the process can proceed as far as a sinus formation over the apex before the condition is discovered at a routine examination.

Commonly the presenting symptom is occasional pain, and, in the very young, this can be interpreted and remembered unreliably by both the parent and child. In some children there is also an element of deliberate denial or misdirection to steer the operator away from a sensitive tooth. Such factors can create diagnostic problems.

Ask direct questions:

Has there been any toothache?
When did it start? Duration?
Where is it located? Area of pain? Exact place?
What makes it better? What makes it worse?
Does it come on spontaneously or as a result of direct stimulation: eating, temperature changes, etc.?
Does it keep the child awake?
Have there been any symptoms of infection, swelling or fever?
Is there any relevant history of trauma?

Examination

General   Is the child ill, toxic, feverish, crying with pain?

Extra-oral   Observation: Look for associated swelling or a red cheek.

Palpation: Gently touch the child. Palpate extra-orally for alveolar swelling (hidden in a chubby cheek) and associated lymph nodes for signs of infection.

Intra-oral   Observation: Is one side of the mouth clean while the other side is dirty? A tooth that is too painful to use, touch or brush is soon covered in plaque.
Ask the child to point to the painful tooth.
Look for cavities or failed restorations in the teeth in the area, check all the teeth on the affected side.
Where the carious marginal ridge has broken away spontaneously in a primary molar tooth pulpal involvement may be expected.
Is the crown discoloured? In an incisor this may indicate previous trauma.
Look for alveolar inflammation, swelling or sinus, both lingually, palatally and buccally. Sinuses can occur at a distance from the affected apex.

Palpation: Is the tooth tender to gentle pressure? Try the adjacent tooth first to accustom the child to the sensation of pressure. Is the affected tooth loose?

Special tests
It is difficult, in most cases, to use and rely upon the results of the conventional pulp testing techniques such as thermal or electrical stimulation: (a) because they may precipitate a painful spasm in the tooth and lose the child's cooperation, and (b) because they are very unreliable in primary teeth that may already be undergoing apical resorption and thus degeneration of the pulpal structure.

Radiograph   Periapical or child's bite-wing views should be obtained (the latter will show the apices of primary molars). Consider taking films of both sides to allow examination and comparison of both the opposing and contralateral teeth for they develop together and, subjected to the same oral environment, may well be carious also.
Examine the radiograph systematically, starting with the crown.

1. The extent of the caries and proximity to the pulp.
2. The condition of existing restorations.
3. The size and condition of the pulp chamber: secondary dentine, calcifications, internal resorption?
4. Roots: shape, internal resorption?
5. Apices: stage of natural resorption, position of apical openings, pathological resorption or delayed resorption?
6. Bone: look for any periapical or bifurcation rarefaction of bone, or pathological widening of the periodontal space or loss of the lamina dura. Check if such rarefactions threaten the tooth germ of the permanent successor.

Direct examination
As treatment proceeds, further information about the depth of caries and the pulp condition will be obtained.

A pulpal exposure will reveal:

1. Normal pulp: red blood flows and is quickly staunched by pressure with a sterile cotton wool pellet.
2. Abnormal pulp: dark red or purple blood flows and it is difficult to obtain haemostasis by pressure with a cotton wool pellet.
3. Dead pulp: the exposure may release pus, a bad odour or reveal dry, gangenous pulp tissue.

A review of choices of treatment procedures

The inexperienced operator is confronted with the confusing abundance of detailed pulp therapy techniques for primary teeth published in recent decades. A standard terminology is not always used, and it is important to discover an author's intended meaning. Experts disagree about the safety and effectiveness of certain medicaments and techniques, and the criteria for success. There is a paucity of controlled scientific evidence to support old empirical methods. Many long-established endodontic drugs have been found to be markedly cytotoxic compared with their antimicrobial effect, e.g. phenol derivatives and protein fixatives. Their continued use requires judgement and care in every case, while the urgent quest for better techniques continues.

1. Pulp capping

Indirect capping

Comment
This technique is rarely used in primary teeth, because ideal conditions for success are difficult to ensure.

Definition
The application of a therapeutic material to an area of infected dentine over the pulp, in a deep cavity where the pulp is not actually exposed.

Indications
Deep cavity that predisposes exposure in a symptomless vital tooth.

Contraindications
A history of spontaneous pain. Clinical or radiographic evidence of pulp pathology.

Materials
Calcium hydroxide (Dycal),

Technique
1. Administer local anaesthetic.
2. Isolate the tooth in case an actual exposure is discovered.
3. Eliminate all peripheral caries leaving a minimal layer overlying the pulp.
4. Prepare the cavity for restoration.
5. Cover the pulpal wall with a thin layer of quick-setting calcium hydroxide material. Consider if a cement lining is needed to resist pressure during subsequent restoration.
6. Restore the tooth permanently.

Direct capping

Definition
The application of a therapeutic material over an exposed vital pulp to induce calcific repair.

Contraindications
This technique is *not* recommended for *primary* teeth because (a) the ideal conditions demanded for success will rarely occur, (b) the application of calcium hydroxide directly to the pulps of primary

teeth generally initiates a process of internal resorption, and (c) the alternative formocresol pulpotomy enjoys a high rate of success.

2. Pulpotomy

Definition
Pulpotomy literally means the amputation of the dental pulp coronal to the dentinocemental junction. However, most authors use the term to indicate partial pulpotomy: the amputation of the entire contents of the pulp chamber leaving the pulp tissue in the root canals undisturbed. (The alternative term 'partial pulpectomy' is deprecated.)

Formocresol pulpotomy

Definition
Amputation of the coronal pulp and treatment of the vital pulp stumps with formocresol.

Indications
An exposed vital pulp that has been symptomless or only transiently hyperaemic.

Contraindications
History of prolonged spontaneous pain, especially at night. Clinical or radiographic signs of apical infection or root resorption. Excessive bleeding from the radicular stumps after amputation, in which case consider devitalizing pulpotomy.

Materials
Formocresol:

Formaldehyde soln (37%) in 60/20 glycerine and water	60%
Cresol	40%

Made up in 10 ml amounts and kept in tightly screwed bottles, it will have a long shelf life.

Recent studies have shown equally good clinical results when this original formocresol formula is used in a 1 in 5 dilution.

Application of formocresol solution to the pulp tissue has been shown to produce three zones of change. The first, in direct contact with the formocresol dressing is a zone of fixation where the cells are no longer active. Next comes the zone of coagulation necrosis with the cells losing some of their microscopic detail. Finally there is the zone of reparative granulation tissue which lies between the necrotic and the normal tissue, and this is thought to be capable of growing back slowly and replacing the necrotic zone. No calcification occurs.

Comment
Recently attention has been focused upon the possible toxic effects of formalin on body tissues both locally and systemically (lungs, kidneys and liver), including mutagenic and carcinogenic effects, when it has been used copiously in a variety of medical treatments and in animal experiments. Medicaments and preparations containing paraformaldehyde or formalin solutions must be used sparingly in root and pulp treatments and not allowed to be extruded beyond the apex, when even a trace may have a local effect on the underlying tooth and bone, and systemically may cause allergic reactions.

Technique
 1. Administer a local anaesthetic.
 2. Isolate the tooth.
 3. Remove all caries except that over the pulp chamber.
 4. Develop a retentive cavity.
 5. Open the pulp chamber widely via the roof ensuring good access and visibility.
 6. Remove the contents of the pulp chamber with a sharp excavator or a large, slowly-rotating, round bur. In the latter case take care not to weaken the walls or floor of the pulp chamber.
 7. Apply a pledget of cotton wool sparingly moistened with formocresol solution to the amputated root stumps and leave it in position for three minutes.
 8. Remove the cotton wool. The amputated ends should have turned black and stopped bleeding. If the bleeding persists proceed to the devitalizing pulpotomy technique.
 9. Cover the floor of the pulp chamber with a stiff mix of cement made up of equal parts of formocresol solution and eugenol combined with zinc oxide powder. Some prefer to avoid the use of further formalin and substitute plain zinc oxide/eugenol cement at this stage.
10. Seal the chamber with conventional lining cement.
11. Restore the tooth permanently.

Treatment of the exposed pulp with a glutaraldehyde solution has been suggested instead of a formalin-based material. A 2 or 5% solution, buffered to an alkaline pH 8.5, with a shelf life of only one week, may be used as in the formocresol technique. It tends to have a haemostatic effect.

Mortal pulpotomy (devitalizing pulpotomy)

Comment
This method was described by Hobson (1970) and advocated by many including Goodman (1985) and Rule (1990), but it has not been so extensively evaluated as the formocresol technique. In the light of the current concern about the danger of apical leakage of formalin products previously mentioned some clinicians have abandoned its use altogether in favour of complete pulpectomy.

Definition
A two-visit devitalizing technique where the medicament is first sealed in direct contact with vital pulp tissue for several days before the coronal pulp is amputated and the pulp stumps covered with antiseptic paste, and the tooth restored. (The term 'mortal' is used here to mean 'subject to or causing death.')

Indications
Where it has not been possible to obtain satisfactory anaesthesia of an exposed vital pulp, or where, following amputation of the coronal pulp, the radicular stumps continue to bleed excessively.

Contraindications
History of prolonged bouts of spontaneous pain. Evidence of periapical infection, abscess or sinus. Wide open apices that may allow the medicament to escape.

Materials
Paraform Paste:

Paraformaldehyde	1.00 g
Lignocaine	0.06 g
Carbowax 1500	1.30 g
Propylene glycol	0.05 g
Carmine	*q.s.* (a sufficient quantity)

Paraformaldehyde slowly releases formalin at body temperature and this disinfectant reacts with proteins, devitalizes and fixes pulp tissue. The lignocaine prevents the patient from feeling discomfort.

The remaining constituents form a coloured vehicle for the active ingredients.

Technique

First visit

1. Administer a local anaesthetic.
2. Isolate the tooth.
3. Remove caries from the tooth and create a retentive cavity.
4. Place a piece (about 1 cmm) of devitalizing paste on a small pledget of cotton wool in close contact (a) with the inadequately anaesthetized pulp exposure (which should be at least 1 mm in diameter) or (b) the amputated bleeding pulp stumps in the fully opened pulp chamber.
5. Cover and seal in the cotton wool dressing with a thin mix of hard-setting cement, avoiding any pressure on the pulp.
6. Ensure that the parent has an analgesic available to give to the child if there is any discomfort during the first night of treatment.

Second visit (after 7–10 days)

1. Check that there has been no history of pain or swelling.
2. Check if the tooth is mobile or if there is any other evidence of apical involvement.
3. No local anaesthetic should be needed for the remaining pulp therapy because the pulp has been devitalized.
4. Isolate the tooth.
5. Remove the cement, the dressing and paste.
6. Where this has not already been achieved proceed to open the pulp chamber widely and remove the dead, fixed coronal tissue.
7. Cover the amputated radicular stumps with a zinc oxide/eugenol paste or the zinc oxide/formocresol/eugenol paste used in the formocresol pulpotomy technique.
8. Seal the pulp chamber with hard-setting cement.
9. Place the permanent restoration.

(Note: Paraform paste must not be left in situ for much longer than the prescribed time of 7–10 days in case formalin escapes via the apex. Failed second visit appointments must be followed-up immediately.)

Non-vital pulpotomy (mummification)

Comment

Ideally a tooth with a non-vital pulp is treated by complete pulpectomy and root filling. For many years, because of the complexity of the root canals in primary molars, mummification has been advocated as an alternative method of treatment of dead radicular pulp tissue, despite a lack of supporting scientific evidence. A certain degree of clinical success has been obtained. Nevertheless, critics of the technique suggest that the method is dangerous because it is not possible to monitor the canal contents, and they prefer to attempt pulpectomy or extract the tooth in such cases.

Definition
Amputation of the coronal pulp tissues of a dead tooth and treatment of the dead pulp stumps by medicaments to mummify them and thus preserve them in an aseptic state. (The term 'mummification' causes confusion. It is used here in the sense that Mummies in the British Museum were preserved *after* death, not devitalized by the process.)

Indications
A symptomless, non-vital tooth.

Contraindications
Medical conditions. History and signs of apical infection.

Materials
Camphorated monochlorphenol (CMP)
Formocresol
Eugenol
Zinc oxide powder

Technique

Stage 1

1. Isolate the tooth.
2. Prepare the cavity for restoration.
3. Open the pulp chamber widely.
4. Remove the contents of the pulp chamber with an excavator or large round bur.
5. Wash away debris with sterile saline and dry with cotton wool.
6. Firmly seal in a dressing of CMP or diluted formocresol on cotton wool placed in the pulp chamber.

Stage 2 (after 7–10 days)

1. Check that the tooth has remained symptomless and has no signs of infection.

3. Remove the dressing.
4. Wash and dry the chamber.
5. Cover the amputated pulp stumps with an antiseptic paste, e.g. zinc oxide/eugenol or the zinc oxide/formocresol/eugenol paste described in the formocresol pulpotomy technique.
6. Seal the pulp chamber with cement.
7. Place the permanent restoration.

3. Pulpectomy

Definition
The complete removal of the pulp from the pulp chamber and root canals to the dentinocemental junction. In primary molars the complex radicular pulp morphology means that complete removal is not mechanically possible.

Indications
Dead pulp. Strong reasons to avoid extraction such as the medical history (e.g. bleeding tendency); space maintenance. This treatment may be considered for a tooth with a sinus or following treatment of an acute abscess by drainage and antibiotic.

Contraindications
Relevant medical history (e.g. heart valve lesions), gross infection with bone loss threatening permanent successor, pathological root resorption, poor patient cooperation.

Materials
Camphorated monochlorphenol (CMP)
Formocresol.
Calcium hydroxide paste

Technique

Stage 1

1. Isolate the tooth.
2. Open the pulp chamber widely.
3. Remove the coronal pulp tissue.
4. Debride the root canals carefully and as completely as possible, gently and repeatedly washing away the debris with sterile saline or dilute hypochlorite solution. Use Hedstrom files (no reamers) but keep short and do not penetrate the apex. The length of the canal can be adequately estimated from the original radiograph. In molars the apical opening lies high on the bifurcation side.

5.   Dry the canal with paper points.
     (Note: In the absence of infection, root filling may be carried
     out at this stage.)
6.   Firmly seal in a dressing of dilute formocresol or CMP on
     cotton wool placed in the pulp chamber.

Stage 2

1.   Check that the tooth has remained symptomless and shows no
     sign of infection.
2.   Isolate the tooth.
3.   Remove the dressing.
4.   Wash and dry the canals.
5.   Fill the canals with a bland resorbable material such as calcium
     hydroxide paste by placing a quantity of the paste in the pulp
     chamber and packing it down the root canals with a plugger.
     Special endodontic syringes have also been suggested for this
     purpose.
6.   Seal the pulp chamber with cement.
7.   Restore the tooth.

Follow-up of a pulp-treated primary tooth

Review the treated tooth at subsequent 4–6 monthly check-ups to
ensure that it remains symptomless. Consider placing a steel crown
to give a weakened tooth extracoronal support. After 6 months take
a radiograph to ensure that there is no evidence of apical pathology.
A devitalized tooth is generally shed early.

Complications
These are rare unless the procedure follows misdiagnosis of the
pulpal condition. Recurrent pain and infection, periapical rarefaction of bone, subclinical deterioration with either pathological or
delayed resorption all indicate the need for extraction.

4. Extraction

Indications

1.   Medical conditions contraindicating pulp therapy.
2.   Crown too broken down to restore.
3.   Tooth is extensively fractured.
4.   More than half the root has already resorbed.
5.   Extensive infection and cellulitis.

6. More than two pulpally exposed teeth present in the mouth.
7. If pulp therapy techniques fail: pain, internal resorption, abscess, delayed exfoliation.

If a tooth has to be extracted consider if a space maintainer is needed or, in the case of multiple extractions, if a denture is required.

Restorative dentistry for young permanent teeth

Permanent molar teeth

Newly erupted six-year-old molars need special consideration. Parents are often unaware that these are permanent teeth and may tend to allow them to be neglected. In addition, in a mouth with a high caries rate, cavities in these teeth, with their immature large pulps may proceed to a point of near-exposure before any discomfort is felt, sometimes even before the tooth is fully erupted. In addition, the broad, flat contact point between the second primary molar and the first permanent molar may allow interproximal caries in both these teeth to proceed undetected by the patient or parent.

Management of the early carious lesion

Incipient lesions
These are defined as minimal or white spot lesions including those on interproximal surfaces where the demineralization is only half the depth of the enamel and where there is no dentine involvement. In cases where there is doubt, for example a stained fissure, then further investigation and fissure treatment or preventive resin restoration will be indicated. It is important to record the site of the incipient lesion and to make sure that it is kept under constant review at subsequent appointments. In addition the patient and/or parent should be shown where the lesion is and encouraged to make every effort to change the intra-oral environment by appropriate dietary choices and restrictions, enhanced oral hygiene with appropriate flossing, together with the use of topical fluorides.

The operator must be ever vigilant to detect 'occult', hidden or 'mushroom' caries where the process penetrates a microscopic pit, fissure or flaw in the enamel, usually on the occlusal surface, to allow extensive symptomless caries to expand into the dentine. When examining radiographs that monitor molar teeth always check the whole enamel surface and the amelodentinal junction, not just the inaccessible contact areas between the teeth.

Preventive Resin Restoration (PRR)

Simonsen (1985) described the technique of minimal caries restoration combined with concomitant sealing of the adjacent caries-susceptible pits and fissures. This means a minimal loss of tooth structure for there is no need for 'extension for prevention' of the cavity.

He describes three types of PRR using this basic technique:

Type 1 PRR.   Where the pit and fissure decay is minimal or where the operator is unsure whether decay is present in a tooth scheduled for fissure sealing. A tiny rosehead bur, size ½, is used to access the caries or to explore the questionable 'sticky' fissure. If the caries does not extend into the dentine, the tiny preparation is kept within the enamel, the tooth is etched and the cavity and adjacent fissures sealed with a filled sealant.

Type 2 PRR.   Where the caries has progressed into the dentine although still confined to a small area. Again the caries is accessed and removed with the smallest burs possible taking care to eliminate possible spread of decay along the amelodentinal junction. After placing a protective base of calcium hydroxide over the dentine, the tooth is etched, an intermediate unfilled resin layer is applied and then the cavity filled with a posterior composite and carried into fissures adjacent to the cavity to seal them. Finally, any remaining fissures on the tooth surface are sealed.

Type 3 PRR.   This is very similar to the Type 2 PRR except that the restorative material is confined to the cavity alone (glass-ionomer cement may be used) and then the restoration and adjacent fissure are sealed with pit and fissure sealant.

Cautious cavity preparation

This is a technique that may be useful for both the primary and permanent teeth where there is extensive and deep caries that threatens pulp exposure. In cases of multiple lesions it may form part of the emergency treatment plan.

The carious lesion is opened and the gross caries is removed by careful instrumentation until the walls of the cavity are clear. The still-carious floor of the cavity is now lined with a calcium hydroxide material and the cavity filled temporarily with a reinforced zinc oxide/eugenol cement. The tooth may be re-opened after some 4 to 6 weeks by which time the formation of secondary dentine, together with a certain degree of hardening of the caries should allow deeper penetration to be made without fear of pulp exposure.

Porcelain veneers

Used to improve the appearance of permanent teeth, particularly maxillary incisors in cases of:

non-vital discoloration
enamel hypocalcification of hypoplasia
fluorosis
tetracycline staining (rare now)
extensive restorations with a poor aesthetic result
fractured teeth
teeth that require recontouring

Some degree of enamel reduction of the tooth is needed. This reduces the extent of overbuild that is necessary with acrylic or composite facing techniques for strength and to mask tooth discoloration. Acrylic or composite facings are adequate in the short term but they become stained within a few months. Porcelain veneers look better, are thinner, resist abrasion, and tend to be less plaque-retentive.

The veneer method may be used for a young patient's immature teeth as an intermediate stage before crowning.

The veneer should be 0.5–0.7 mm thick constructed to cover the labial aspect of the prepared maxillary incisor tooth and will be luted to remaining enamel surface with composite resin. The veneer is extended to the contact area approximally, but preferably kept coronal to the gingival margin. The incisal margin of the veneer may be confined entirely on the labial aspect of the incisal edge or, alternatively, may be wrapped over it, the latter condition makes the positioning of the final restoration easier and, where necessary, allows incisal lengthening.

The fit surface of the veneer is etched with acid or sandblasted and then treated with a silane coupling agent. This agent bonds to the silicate of the porcelain while the contained methacrylate group is free to bond with the composite layer which is turn is attached to the tooth enamel.

Preparation   The tooth is restored if necessary. The enamel is reduced using a round-ended diamond bur, e.g. HiDi 504. Depth cuts should be made initially to guide the extent of enamel reduction and thus avoid exposure of dentine. A finishing line should be developed near the gingival margin. The amount of reduction may depend upon the necessity to mask the colour of the tooth or to recontour it. The path of insertion is from the labial and slightly incisal direction. Polishing strips may be used to ensure separation between the teeth.

Impression   A retraction cord is used to displace the gingivae where necessary. The impression may be taken in a special tray using a silicone impression material. If the margin of the tray is kept to a minimum on the palatal aspect the impression may be removed in a more labial direction.

Shade selection is made with a porcelain shade guide, taking note of any special characteristics to be added.

Temporary coverage, where needed, may be with composite on the unetched enamel, for this can be chipped off readily at a later stage.

Try-in   The prepared fitting surface of the veneer must not be touched when it is returned from the laboratory. The shade is checked and then the tooth and the adjacent teeth are isolated (for colour and contour matching), preferably with rubber dam. The tooth is cleaned with pumice and water or an oil and glycerine-free polishing agent. The gingivae must not be abraded or the bleeding will interfere with the veneer attachment. However, any gingival oozing can be controlled by the application of retraction cord. The veneer is tried on the clean and dry tooth, checking the colour and the margins. Tight contacts may be gently reduced with a diamond disc or stone. The colour of the veneer can be modified even at this stage by the use of shaded composites. If these are to be tried into the veneer the latter should have the etched surface treated with the silane coupling agent and unfilled resin before the light-cure composite is placed in it.

Bonding   The adjacent teeth are isolated with a matrix strip moulded around the palatal surface of the prepared tooth. Any exposed dentine must be protected. The enamel is now etched and the tooth washed and dried. Then the etch is checked for adequacy. If it has not already been done the silane priming agent is applied to the porcelain fit surface. This is followed by a small amount of the unfilled resin which is dispersed over the fit surface with a gentle air-jet. Next a thin layer of composite it applied to the veneer avoiding air-bubbles. These manipulations of light-cured resin and composite should be carried out in a low-light level to reduce the chance of premature curing.

The veneer is slid into place on the tooth. Enough composite should have been used to cause excess material to be extruded from the margins of the veneer. The shade should be checked again, for on rare occasions, even at this late stage it may be necessary to remove the veneer and use another colour of composite. If all is well the veneer may be 'tacked' into place with a 10-sec burst of the curing light before the marginal excess is carefully removed with a probe and with unwaxed dental floss in the difficult contact areas. Once everything appears to be satisfactory the composite is then completely light cured, allowing time for the light to penetrate the porcelain. Some confident operators are willing to use self-cured composite materials to lute the veneer to the tooth. They claim that it is difficult to ensure adequate light-curing via the thickness of the porcelain veneer. There are also composites that are said to combine the light-cure and self-cure properties once the curing has been initiated by the light source.

Finishing   Once the composite has set any further excess is removed with a scalpel or flame finishing burs. The occlusion is checked with articulating paper and any necessary adjustments to the porcelain contour made with diamond instruments. Finally the margins and any adjustment areas are polished with soflex discs and polishing strips.

The patient is instructed about maintaining good oral hygiene particularly in the area of the veneer and a mouth guard should be provided if they take part in certain sports activities that are liable to put the teeth at risk.

Minimal or non-preparation bridges

These bridges can be constructed to replace lost permanent anterior teeth and thus avoid the need for a removable appliance. They are very useful for young patients. A simple bridge can be made attaching the pontic via metal attachments to the surfaces of adjacent teeth using the acid-etch composite technique. Minimal preparation may be needed to allow an unrestricted insertion path.

The Rochette bridge is retained by undercut perforations in the metal of the attachment flanges through which the composite can flow. The fitting surfaces of the perforated flanges are sand blasted in the laboratory to remove all oxide and to improve the adaption of the composite. If the bridge needs to be removed later, then the composite can be drilled away to facilitate this.

The Maryland bridge has no perforations, but the fitting surfaces are specially treated to produce an etched retentive surface similar to etched enamel. The attachment flanges can be thinner because there are no perforations to weaken them.

For further details of routine restoration of permanent teeth the reader should consult a standard textbook of adult conservative dentistry.

Endodontic treatment for young permanent teeth

Pulpal involvement in young permanent teeth usually arises as a result of deep caries or trauma, but very occasionally exposure occurs during injudicious preparation of the tooth for restoration.

Newly-erupted permanent teeth still have large pulp chambers and open apices.

Deep caries in a molar tooth indicates the need to assess the whole mouth very carefully. For example, gross caries in one six-year-old molar may be accompanied by equally deep carious cavities in the other contemporary molars. Periapical radiographs, an OPT view may be required before deciding whether to restore or extract teeth with a doubtful long-term prognosis.

Pulpal diagnosis

Follows the conventional sequence:

History: General, Dental, Tooth, Pulp.

Examination: Observation, Palpation.
   Special Tests:
   Transillumination. Radiographs.
   Depending upon the child's age and ability to respond reliably, thermal and electric tests for pulp vitality can be made.
Direct Examination.

As described in the Primary Tooth section, further clinical information about pulpal normality, abnormality or death will be obtained as treatment proceeds.

Choices of treatment procedures

1. Direct pulp capping
2. Vital pulpotomy
3. Apexification (induced apical closure)

1. Direct pulp capping
(See also Cautious Cavity Preparation and Indirect Pulp Capping.)

Definition
The application of a therapeutic material over an exposed vital pulp to induce calcific repair.

Indications
This technique is only recommended for vital, asymptomatic, non-infected pulps of *permanent* teeth with a small, recent exposure not exceeding 2 mm in diameter.

Contraindications
Exposures of more than 2 mm diameter. Prolonged exposure (over 6 hours) to the infective environment of the mouth. Carious exposure surrounded by infected dentine. Symptoms and signs of pulpal pathology. A closed apex reduces the blood supply and may affect the chance of success, but is not itself a contraindication.

Materials
Calcium hydroxide preparations (e.g. Dycal).

Technique

1. Isolate the tooth (preferably before anticipated exposure).
2. Wash the exposed surface with saline solution and then protect it with a small pledget of cotton wool moistened with saline.
3. Prepare a retentive cavity.
4. Remove the cotton wool and cover the exposure with calcium hydroxide preparation.
5. Seal over the calcium hydroxide with a cement base. Avoid pressure.
6. Restore the tooth.

Follow-up
Review the tooth in a month or in the event of pain (which may indicate the onset of pulpal inflammation). The tooth should remain asymptomatic and respond normally to pulp vitality tests. Radiographs taken after six months may show evidence of repair by the formation of a calcific bridge under the calcium hydroxide layer.

Complications
Slow onset of pulpal necrosis requiring further endodontic treatment.

2. Vital pulpotomy

Definition
Amputation of the coronal pulp and treatment of the vital pulp stumps with calcium hydroxide.

Indications
This technique is only recommended in permanent teeth with large

exposures (over 2 mm in diameter), with minimal pulpal inflammation or infection judged to remain confined to the pulp chamber only and leaving the pulp tissue in the root canals unaffected, and with open apices.

Contraindications
Clinical or radiographic indications of periapical infection. Persistent haemorrhage from the amputated pulp stumps. Non-vital pulp. Pus in the root canals.

Technique

1. Administer local anaesthetic.
2. Isolate the tooth.
3. Prepare a retentive cavity.
4. Open the roof of the pulp chamber widely.
5. Remove the pulp tissue from the coronal pulp chamber.
6. Assess the condition of the pulp stumps.
7. Wash the chamber clean with saline solution and dry with sterile cotton wool pledgets.
8. Cover the stumps with calcium hydroxide/sterile water paste pressed into place with cotton wool.
9. Seal over the calcium hydroxide with a cement base. Avoid pressure.
10. Restore the tooth.

Follow-up
Review the tooth in a month's time or immediately if pain is experienced. Take radiographs at six-monthly intervals to monitor the growth and closure of the root apex. It may be possible to see evidence of the calcified bridge formed under the calcium hydroxide layer.

Complications
Rarely, pulpal necrosis and apical infection.

3. Apexification (induced apical closure)

Definition
Inducing apical closure in a young permanent tooth which has a chronically infected root canal. (Success depends upon the ability of the epithelial sheath of Hertwig, surrounding the forming apical tissues of the tooth, to continue to organize the apex formation despite the occurrence of recent local infection.)

Indications
An immature permanent tooth, usually an incisor, with an infected root canal and an incompletely formed apex, where it is considered important to avoid extraction.

Comment
A successful outcome obviates the need for apical surgery and retrograde root filling.

Contraindications
Medical reasons for avoiding root canal therapy. Clinical and radiographic indications of gross apical infection and bone loss.

Technique

Stage 1
Acute infection must be resolved by drainage and/or antibiotic therapy preoperatively.

1. Administer a local anaesthetic.
2. Isolate the tooth.
3. Open the pulp chamber to allow instrument access to the root canal.
4. Cautiously remove debris and pulp tissue from the root canal with files taking care not to penetrate too far, remaining 2 mm short of the apical tissues.
5. Wash out the debris with saline solution.
6. Dry the canal with paper points.
7. Dress the canal:
   (a) If considered to be badly infected, with beechwood creosote or camphorated monochlorphenol (CMP) on cotton wool.
   (b) With calcium hydroxide paste, e.g. Hypocal which is presented in a syringe.
8. Seal the root canal with cement.

Stage 2: after 7–10 days

1. Assess the tooth for signs of residual infection which means a further period with a new dressing.
2. Isolate the tooth.
3. Open the root canal and remove the dressing. Wash out the calcium hydroxide; it does not set hard.
4. Assess the root canal and decide if a further period with a dressing is needed.
5. Fill the root canal with calcium hydroxide paste.
6. Seal the root canal.

Follow-up
Review the tooth immediately if there is any pain. Take radiographs at six-monthly intervals to monitor apical development and closure. When closure has occurred wash out the calcium hydroxide and proceed with conventional root canal filling procedures. In some cases the open apex repair is confined to the production of a calcified barrier or plug that seals the root canal but does not give the normal root apex. Nevertheless this is still a successful outcome.

Complications
Continual apical infection and bone loss. The 'blunderbuss' apical shape of an immature permanent tooth makes apical surgery difficult. In some cases extraction may have to be considered.

Chapter 7

Minor oral surgery

In general practice nearly all minor oral surgery for children is concerned with carrying out dental extractions and the treatment of dental infections.

Any surgery for children presents the operator with special challenges compared with treating the adult. The child's tissues are more delicate, the anatomy and the general metabolism differ when considering drugs, anaesthesia, haemorrhage and the care of infection; the mouth is smaller; and the child is more likely to externalize his fears and anxieties.

Treatment planning

This is based on a comprehensive medical and dental history and examination, radiographs and a sound diagnosis.

The operator must decide if he is competent to carry out the operation; he must consider if he has the confidence, experience, surgery facilities, instruments and supporting staff to ensure success. If there is any doubt then he should refer the child to a specialist centre or hospital.

Referral to hospital for in-patient treatment should also be recommended for:

Complicated extractions
Anaesthetic problems
Behavioural problems
Severe handicaps
Medical or drug reaction problems
Bleeding tendencies
Very severe infections
Maxillofacial injuries
Tumours and neoplasms

Choice of anaesthetic

The first consideration is to decide if the proposed operation will require local or general anaesthesia. Provided that the child, the parent and the operator share mutual confidence, the bulk of minor oral surgery of short duration is carried out under local anaesthesia. Some children may benefit from the addition of a sedative pre-medication or relative analgesia.

A general anaesthetic will be indicated for prolonged operations, multiple or potentially difficult extractions and those requiring noisy bone removal, for abscesses and cases where local analgesia is not appropriate, and for very young, very apprehensive or mentally handicapped patients.

Preparation for surgery

Timing
A decision has to be made about the timing of the operation. Emergencies involving haemorrhage, pain, severe infection, etc. have to be dealt with immediately while other operations may be carried out electively after a short interval of a few days.

Parent

Make sure that the parent is fully informed about what you want to do because then:

1. They can give informed consent to surgery and persuade you to proceed, rather than feeling unwillingly pressured into agreement.
2. They can support the child more if their own fear of the unknown has been taken from them.
3. They can help during the recovery period after the child has left the surgery.
4. They won't transfer any guilt about the need for extractions, for example, into anger and resentment of the operator, should a complication arise.

Preparing the child

Although the operator must take into account the age of the child there is an element of controversy about how best to prepare it for any kind of surgery. Some authorities, usually dentists, suggest that there should not be a long gap between the decision and the operation because this will give the child time to worry and to build up a nervous tension and as a result it will be less cooperative. Another view suggests that the child needs time to come to terms with the loss of a valuable tooth and that a period of up to a week before the operation is more appropriate. Unnecessary urgency might also make the child more apprehensive for all future dental appointments if he thinks that he can be subjected to surgery at a moment's notice!

Whichever course the operator chooses the child should certainly be prepared mentally for surgery by giving him a simple explanation of what is to happen, and every means of emotional support and sympathy from then on. If he is told nothing at all until the moment of general anaesthetic induction, for example, he may understandably imagine that the uncomfortable effects of elective surgery are some kind of punishment.

Extraction of children's teeth

General preparation

Before the patient arrives, the surgery and instruments should be prepared. The operator should review the patient's records and think through the sequences he is about to undertake.

The forceps to be used are generally the operator's personal choice. For primary teeth small forceps with smaller tips can approximate to the tooth size better than adult forceps and are less obvious when held in the hand.

e.g. Ash Lustra forceps:

No. 37:	Children's Upper incisors and canines
No. 39:	Upper molars
No. 123:	Lower teeth and roots
No. 138:	Upper teeth and roots

Contingency instruments should also be prepared in case a simple extraction proves difficult, e.g. when extracting a permanent tooth:

Scalpel, periosteal elevator, surgical burs and handpiece, elevators, rongeurs, bone file, needle holder, scissors, sutures (cat-gut resorbable for children, black silk), sterile packs.

Extraction of primary teeth

This presents special problems to the operator:

1.   The crowns of the primary teeth are smaller, the roots of the

molar teeth are divergent, and the mouth is smaller. This affects the choice of forceps.
2. The roots are very fine, brittle and, during part of their life-cycle, may be resorbing or ankylosed.
3. The primary teeth are in close approximation to the underlying permanent tooth germ and these are at risk during the extraction of their predecessors.
4. The bone structure of the jaws is generally smaller and more delicate.

Simple extractions

1. Take radiographs first to assess the tooth and adjacent structures.
2. Inject the local anaesthetic agent and wait for it to work. Test the effect with a probe.
3. Sit the conscious child up when extracting under local anaesthesia to avoid him swallowing or inhaling the tooth if it is dropped into his numb mouth.
4. Get the dental surgery assistant to stabilize the patient's head.
5. Apply the forceps and press up apically to gain a good grip on root, but don't drive them in too forcibly.
6. Upper primary incisors and canines have straight, cone-shaped roots, and may be loosened by rotating back and forth around the long axis.
7. Upper primary molars: apply force palatally first and then buccally. When movement has been obtained then loosen the tooth with further buccopalatal movements.
8. Lower primary incisors and canines: apply force first labially and then lingually and loosen the tooth with only labiolingual movements. These teeth are not conical but elliptical.
9. Lower primary molars: drive the forceps to grip the mesial root. Apply force buccally first then loosen the tooth with buccolingual movements.
10. Put tooth out of sight for the moment.
11. Squeeze socket between your thumb and finger to replace the buccal plate and give child a firm gauze pad to bite on.

(Note: In the event that a primary tooth root fractures during extraction, unless the retained root is loose and easily visible, it is best not to attempt to remove it. Commonly these kind of fragments move to the surface over the course of the next few weeks and are quietly exfoliated. Certainly digging for root fragments with an elevator will put the permanent tooth in danger. Inform the parent and follow up the fragment radiographically.)

Extraction of permanent teeth

The reader is referred to a standard oral surgery textbook.

After care

Try to keep the haemorrhage and blood-stained packs out of sight. Avoid rinsing the mouth but when the child spits out have a lot of water running in the spittoon to conceal any bleeding which can upset some children. Do not allow the child to leave the surgery before the bleeding has stopped.

The extracted tooth is most valuable to the child and whenever possible it must be washed, dried and returned to the owner. The legend of a 'tooth fairy' who replaces the tooth with a silver coin has traditionally helped generations of younger children to accept, and come to terms psychologically with their loss.

Post-extraction instructions
(Give the patient printed instructions about after care.)

'No vigorous rinsing.
No violent exercise for 24 hours.
No very hot or cold food or drink for 24 hours.
Eat with care.
Protect anaesthetized parts.
Tomorrow, keep the mouth very clean and use frequent hot salt water mouthwashes.
If there is any post-extraction bleeding, clean the mouth with cold water, bite firmly over the socket on a clean handkerchief, sit still and don't move the pack for 10 minutes. If the bleeding cannot be stopped in one hour ring this emergency telephone number.'
(Note: The operator should make sure that an analgesic is available for use at home in case the child experiences after-pain when the local anaesthetic wears off.)

Post-extraction haemorrhage
May be the result of not following the instructions. In the surgery: Wash the mouth gently with cold water to remove blood clots. Identify the bleeding point and apply a pressure pack. Get the patient to sit still, biting on the pack for 10 minutes. Reassure them. Decide if a suture over the socket will help. In the rare event that these attempts fail and the bleeding persists take steps to get the child to hospital immediately. Remember that a child is more vulnerable to the effects of blood loss than the adult. In hospital the child will have blood tests, including bleeding and clotting time, to speed the diagnosis of any previously unsuspected bleeding

tendency and there is the back-up of hospitalization and transfusion if necessary.

Acute dental abscess

This is characterized by inflammation, swelling, pain, fever, malaise and usually arises from dental apical infection.

In children the apices of the teeth lie at different levels in relationship to the fascial spaces than in the adult and thus acute apical infections tend to be less contained and more likely to cause extensive facial swelling and cellulitis.

Infection spreading towards the orbit and causing swelling involving the eyelids carries the risk of subsequent cavernous sinus thrombosis if the infection passes backwards via the infraorbital vessels into the skull.

Deep infection extending into the submaxillary spaces may cause trismus and threaten the airway.

Treatment

All acute infections of this kind demand rapid treatment, vigilant observation and frequent follow-up until the condition has been resolved.

1. Establish drainage
Alternatives:

(a) Open the tooth to drain via the root canal.
(b) Incise a pointing abscess in the sulcus.
(c) Extract the tooth to allow drainage via the socket. In some cases consider if drainage via the root canal and antibiotic therapy should come before the extraction to prevent further dispersal of the infection.

2. Remove cause of infection
Extract the infected tooth or consider the alternative possibility of future pulp therapy, root canal therapy or apicectomy.

3. Supportive treatment
Analgesics and for minor, contained infections without cellulitis, local heat in the form of frequent hot salt water mouthwashes. Make sure a feverish child is drinking plenty of fluids and resting.

4. Antibiotic therapy

Prescribe a course of a broad-spectrum antibiotic immediately. If the infection is very severe try to get a sample of pus for laboratory examination of the organism's sensitivity to particular antibiotics in case the drug prescribed is not the most effective.

Chronic dental abscess

In a fit child, neglected subclinical pulp pathology in a primary tooth may result in a chronic apical infection relieved by a localized discharging sinus. This condition is not always painful and may be concealed or unnoticed by the child. Chronic apical infection can delay normal primary root resorption or may extend to threaten the forming succeeding tooth and lead to enamel hypoplasia. A radiograph will allow the operator to assess periapical pathology and to decide if the tooth may be retained after pulp therapy or if it should be extracted.

Chapter 8

Shared orthodontic–paedodontic problems

Premature loss of primary teeth

The effects can depend on the child's age, the particular tooth and the presence of any crowding. The premature loss of a tooth tends to exaggerate existing problems.

Incisors. Early loss may have little effect on the occlusion, but will affect the child's speech and aesthetic appearance. Where there is already marked crowding, space will be lost.

Canines. Early loss may allow crowded incisors to take up space and also the teeth distal to the canine to drift forwards leaving little space for the permanent canine to erupt into later. Loss of one canine can result in a shift of the centre line. This is difficult to correct later and may be a reason for balancing the extraction by removing the other canine from that arch.

Molars. Loss of the 1st molar results in space loss for the premolars but relief for incisor crowding, and again the need for a possible balancing extraction should be considered. Early loss of the 2nd molar allows forward drifting of the 1st permanent molar to trespass into the premolar space. The fitting of a space maintainer should be considered.

Space maintainers can be made in several ways. As the name suggests their function is to prevent teeth from drifting into a premature space in the arch. These may be teeth adjacent to the gap or opposing teeth from the other jaw. The appliance may be removable, e.g. in the form of a small acrylic plate with clasps, or fixed, e.g. a stainless steel crown or an orthodontic circumferential band with a wire loop welded to it to contact the next tooth across the space. Such appliances demand good oral hygiene and regular review appointments to ensure that they are working properly and are removed immediately the permanent tooth erupts into the space.

Loss of permanent teeth

Again the effects depend upon the age of the patient, the tooth involved and the presence of crowding, but now the long-term oral hygiene and restorative prognoses must be borne in mind.

Incisors. These are usually lost as a result of trauma. (Protruding incisors demand early orthodontic treatment to reduce this risk.) In some crowded cases the tooth loss represents a space gain which can be used by the orthodontist in controlled realignment of the remaining teeth. Teeth adjacent to the missing incisor may be moved or tilted by orthodontic means to allow subsequent grinding and/or the addition of acid-etch restorations or the construction of crowns to restore the teeth to good appearance.

Sometimes in uncrowded cases it is better to maintain the space by constructing a partial denture with spurs to prevent tooth tilting. In appropriate conditions an avulsed tooth might be reimplanted as a space maintainer. Later an adhesive bridge may be constructed if the roots of the remaining teeth are suitable. If the space is neglected and no treatment is given, the remaining incisor teeth can quickly tilt into positions that make subsequent aesthetic restoration extremely difficult.

Canines. These teeth erupt late into the mouth and gain the benefit of previously learned dental care. They are thus rarely lost due to dental caries in childhood. Their extraction is usually for orthodontic reasons where they are located far from the correct position, e.g. impacted in such a way that even surgical repositioning of the tooth into the arch is not possible.

Premolars. These may sometimes be extracted for orthodontic reasons, e.g. in serial extractions, to create space for realignment of teeth where there is a disproportion between the teeth and the jaws. Premature loss for other reasons will tend to allow teeth posterior to the canine to drift forward to take up the space.

Molars. The loss of a 1st permanent molar tooth is never ideal from an orthodontic point of view, and when a single molar is at risk every measure should be considered to avoid extraction. However, poor mineralization or deep caries and periapical infection may mean that the tooth has a poor long-term prognosis and that early loss is inevitable.

Loss of this tooth may result in mesioangular tilting of the 2nd molar (with some rotation around the palatal root in the upper), distal drifting of crowded teeth anterior to the space with resultant centre-line shift and, in some cases, the failure of space closure.

In order to mitigate these problems:

1. Assess the prognosis of 1st permanent molars as early as possible (7 years of age) and make a provisional long-term treatment plan. This may include the temporary restoration to preserve them until the optimum time for extraction.
2. Take radiographs to ensure that the other teeth are present and developing properly.
3. The most favourable time to extract the 1st permanent molar is at about 9½ years of age when the 2nd molar development has just reached the root bifurcation and the tooth is still covered in bone. This will allow time for the position of the 2nd molar to improve before eruption.
4. If the extraction of the 1st permanent molar must be undertaken earlier, there is less tendency for distal drifting if the unerupted 2nd premolar is still embraced by the roots of the 2nd primary molar.
5. If the permanent 2nd molars are already erupting they will tend to tilt if the 1st molar extraction cannot be delayed until they are in occlusion and thus locked in position.
6. In an uncrowded case the loss of an upper 1st molar on its own may still allow a satisfactory result. Loss of a lower 1st molar may require a compensating extraction of the opposing upper molar to allow a good buccal segment relationship to develop.
7. The extraction of one molar should not be contemplated in isolation. For example, consider:
   (a) The condition and prognosis of the other molars.
   (b) Malocclusion or crowding tendencies that may require an orthodontic opinion before extraction, and appliance therapy later.
   (c) The possible need for compensating or balancing extractions.
   (d) Dental health education to preserve the remaining teeth and prevent further tooth loss.

Space analysis/arch measurement

Decisions about potential crowding may be assisted by using one of several published methods for predicting the mesiodistal width of unerupted permanent canines and premolars in mixed dentition patients, based on both measurements from radiographs and the sizes of erupted teeth (Nance, 1947; Hickson and Oldfather, 1958; Tanaka and Johnson, 1974).

The simplest of these methods is that of Tanaka and Johnson which uses the width of the erupted permanent mandibular incisors to predict the width of the permanent canines and premolars using the formula: upper—half the width of the incisors plus 11.00 mm: lower—half the width of the incisors plus 10.5 mm. Such estimates are used together with clinical judgement about other aspects of the mouth to make decisions about treatment for a particular patient.

Ectopic eruption

The eruption of the upper 1st permanent molar is relatively commonly impeded when it becomes locked in place by the upper 2nd primary molar, occasionally causing distal resorption of that tooth. The condition is seen clinically or on a radiograph. The condition should be kept under observation; half of these cases should correct themselves otherwise they will require orthodontic treatment.

Retained teeth

The primary tooth may be dead or there may be a malposition or non-development of the successor. A retained tooth may cause deflected eruption of the permanent successor. After checking that there is a successor the tooth should be extracted.

Submerging molar

This usually happens due to ankylosis of the root, generally of a primary molar. The periodontal membrane is obliterated and the tooth fuses directly to the bone. The aetiology is obscure. As growth proceeds the tooth falls below the occlusal level and the adjacent teeth tilt in over it. The necessary extraction of such a tooth can be quite difficult.

Habits

It is well known that thumb or fingersucking habits can be the cause of malocclusion. Many children start these habits at an early age and they are especially prone to continue them at times of stress or at night when they are tired and ready for sleep. Generally the habit stops spontaneously at about six years of age. However, it may continue later and by the age of nine years a child needs help to overcome the habit.

At the outset it is important to evaluate why the child has continued the habit; it may be under considerable psychological stress which requires investigation and easing. The condition will not be overcome by teasing, humiliating or browbeating the culprit. The child has to make the decision to want to stop the activity for himself and then be shown how to break the habit. This can usually be achieved by a simple reminder: the child can wear a glove on the offending hand at night, or stick a protruding length of sticking plaster onto the digit or even to paint the fingernail with a bitter tasting varnish. Whichever method is chosen, the child feels that he is in charge and able to choose to do it, rather than being forced by well-meaning adults. In recalcitrant cases generous rewards for good behaviour or hypnosis may be successful in breaking the habit.

Oral hygiene

Most orthodontists require the child to reduce its plaque score to an acceptable level (say less than 10%) before they are willing to place an appliance in that mouth. Any orthodontic appliance, fixed or removable, or a denture, acts as a potential plaque trap and requires vigilant oral hygiene supervision by all who see the child.

Developmental problems

In cases where there are anomalies of oral structures, e.g. cleft palate, or in the form, size or number of teeth, the combination of surgical, restorative and orthodontic skills will be required.

The team approach is recommended in the care of the cleft palate case—the surgeon, the orthodontist, the paedodontist, the speech therapist, the oral hygienist, the dental health educator.

Chapter 9

Traumatic injuries to the teeth

Traumatic injury to a child's teeth can be a very upsetting and frightening event for both the child and its parents. Where the injury involves disfiguring fracture or loss of the maxillary incisors the injury can have an emotional effect out of proportion to the seriousness of the injury. Formerly extrovert children may become self-conscious about their appearance and try not to smile.

At the same time the accident often presents the busy dental surgeon with an emergency that has to be fitted into the already crowded day's schedule and it is important that he does not, in his haste, neglect a thorough examination and assessment of the injury if he is to give the best and most appropriate treatment.

Approximately 30% of primary and 29% of permanent teeth will be traumatized to a varying degree (Andreasen, 1981). By the age of 12 years some 10% of children will present for treatment although many more never report the injury. Some 70% of these injuries involve the upper central incisors. Boys injure their teeth more often than girls and 2–4 and 8–10 years of age are the peak periods for these injuries to occur. The accidents also appear to be more common in the spring and early summer.

Predisposing causes include such things as: protruding teeth with no lip coverage; bad eye sight; slow responses; hyperactivity; physical handicap; participation in active contact sports; learning to walk; big new shoes; weak teeth; grossly carious or heavily-filled teeth.

Describing the causes: accidents that traumatize the teeth may occur in many varied ways, including falls, fights, sports injuries, bicycle accidents and so on, as well as in bizarre and shaming ways. Remember that unless the injury has occurred on the sports field or in heroic circumstances, it is not uncommon for the child, fearing punishment, to minimize the event. 'I fell up the stairs', 'I walked into a door', rather than 'I fell from a first storey window', etc. Don't allow the injury to be minimized too much for a direct blow hard enough to fracture a tooth can be likened to being hit with a carpenter's hammer.

Seriously injured children, for example those involved in road traffic accidents, may not remember the events due to the amnesic effects of concussion.

In some cases sinister reasons, such as glue-sniffing, intoxication, drugs or non-accidental injury can also lead to problems in gaining the correct history of the injury.

Emergency care/examination

Traumatic injury to the teeth should be treated as an emergency. The child should be seen as soon as possible, certainly on the same day. A discussion with the parent or teacher on the telephone about the injury can in no way replace the direct examination of the child.

When the child first arrives in the surgery it is important to make an assessment of his general condition. Although a loose or broken tooth may be the most obvious symptom it is important for the dentist to review the child's overall condition as quickly as possible to ensure that a more serious injury of higher priority has not been overlooked.

Confirm that there is no serious haemorrhage or impeded respiratory function and that the child is fully conscious. Check quickly if there is any severe pain or injury elsewhere in the body.

Deal with urgent problems, e.g. if a tooth has been knocked out early reimplantation is vital.

Then, move calmly and reassuringly through the usual systems of history taking and examination.

History

Name
Address
Date of birth (see Note 1 below)
Date of examination

Previous medical history (PMH) (2)
Patient complains of (C/O) (3)
    General
    Dental

History of the injury:

Date and time (4)
How and where the accident occurred (5)

Did the child lose consciousness? (6)
Any amnesia, headache, vomiting?
Is the injury confined to the teeth and jaws? (7)
Previous history of injury to the teeth and jaws? (8)

Notes on history taking

1. Date of birth. Gives an idea of the stage of tooth development.
2. Review the previous medical history, as usual. Identify conditions that may affect the treatment plan, e.g. epilepsy, handicap, bleeding tendency, heart valve lesions.
    (Special note: Determine and record the child's tetanus status.)
3. Patient complains of:
    General: Ask 'How do you feel?' and listen closely. Responses such as 'Headache, blocked or runny nose, sick, hard to breathe, hurts when I breathe, etc.' all require further investigation.
    Dental: Patients are usually more concerned with the pain from soft tissue injury. The injured tooth seems numb.
    'Sharp edges; it hurts when I touch the tooth; the tooth looks funny' are common complaints.
4. Date and time of injury. Important for such things as the decision to re-implant an avulsed tooth, or to cap an exposed pulp.
5. How and where the accident occurred. This allows assessment of the direction and force of the injury.
    Outdoor injuries may be contaminated with soil and prophylaxis against tetanus infection must be considered.
6. Did the child lose consciousness? Does he suffer amnesia, headache, sleepiness or vomiting? All are indications of a possible severe cranial injury that will require further investigation in hospital, e.g. examination by a doctor and cranial radiographs.
7. Is the injury confined to the teeth and jaws? This allows a further chance to review the possibility of injury elsewhere in the body, concealed by the clothes, e.g. ribs, abdomen, limbs etc. A busy dentist must not focus his attention on the teeth too early.
8. Previous history of injury to the teeth and jaws. An accident-prone child may have suffered a confusing previous injury to the same teeth, e.g. a prior broken root.

On examination

General physical condition

Does this child need to be referred directly to a local casualty department?

Head and neck

Extra-oral   (record injuries, cuts, bruises, possible foreign bodies, etc.)

Face

Eyes Sight, eye movement.

Nose Check possible fracture, bleeding, cerebrospinal fluid leaking (CSF) from basal skull fracture.

Ears Hearing, bleeding or CSF leakage.

Lips

Skin sensation (bony displacement injury may affect nerve tracts. If necessary check through the cranial nerves functions).

Movements: Face, tongue, jaws.

Skull

Stand behind and above the child and look for any gross deformity of structure.

Palpate over vault checking for swellings, steps, deformities, depressions, cuts, etc.

Palpate the main facial outlines: orbits, zygomatic arches, condyles and TMJs, mandible. Check mandibular movement path.

Intra-oral

Identify traumatized teeth, but check them all.

Look for:

Displacement of teeth.
Occlusion—any derangement.
Alveolus—any bruising or laceration of overlying mucosa.
Gingival bleeding.
Mobility of teeth.
Tenderness of tooth to pressure.
Colour of tooth.
Caries.
Previous restoration.

Classify the fracture as soon as possible.
Draw a diagram of the fracture as soon as possible.

Special tests

1. Vitality tests
Test a contralateral undamaged tooth first to obtain a baseline of reaction. Avoid excessive levels of stimulation when examining a possibly concussed tooth.

(a) Thermal tests. Usually tested with cold: Liquid ethyl chloride is more consistently cold evaporating from a whole cotton wool roll than from a pledget. A piece or pencil of ice is generally more acceptable and is odourless.

(b) Electric pulp test. Vitality tests made soon after injury may not induce a response from a concussed tooth. Do not assume the tooth is non-vital but arrange further tests after 7–10 days. However, an early diminished response means damage of some degree and the pulp has to be monitored regularly in future.

2. Transillumination
The light source can range from that reflected by a mouth mirror to the use of more sophisticated fibreoptic equipment with a choice of different coloured light filters ranging from plain white to green and yellow. Light transmitted through the tooth can give direct evidence of pulpal damage resulting in bleeding into dentine, and reveal severe enamel crazing invisible by direct light yet indicative of severe disruption.

3. Radiography
Every traumatized tooth must be examined radiographically. The examination is not complete without it. Consider if adjacent teeth should be examined in this way as well.
In cases where the root may be fractured two radiographs are taken to show the tooth from different angles to aid diagnosis.
Reduced exposure radiographs may be taken of soft tissues of lip or tongue where there is a suspicion that tooth or foreign body fragments might have been driven into wounds.
More extensive radiographs will be required if there is a possible fracture of the jaws or skull.
Always examine every radiograph systematically and take care to check the whole film every time (adjacent teeth, bone, pathology, etc.).

Classification

Many classifications of traumatic injuries to the teeth have been proposed including those of Bennett (1963), Ellis and Davey (1970), the World Health Organisation's Application of the International Classification of Diseases to Dentistry and Stomatology ICA-DA, 2nd edn (1978), and those described in Andreasen (1981) and Hargreaves *et al.* (1981). Such classifications are either descriptive or numeric lists, but as O'Donnell and Wei (1988) point out there is no real standardization. Although lists may differ in detail and complexity it is important to choose one that is easy to remember and leads to a systematic approach to the subject for busy clinicians and fraught examination candidates. The present classification is based simplistically on aspects of all those mentioned above, and describes the possible effects of trauma on the dental and associated tissues from the tip of the tooth to the apex and beyond.

Classification of traumatic injuries to the teeth and supporting structure

Tooth

Class 0   Intact: no fracture, but enamel cracked

Class 1   Enamel fractured

Class 2   Dentine fractured

Class 3   Pulp exposed

        Crown/root fracture ⎫ involves
        Pulp not exposed ⎬ classes
        Pulp exposed   ⎭ $2, 4 \pm 3$

Class 4   Root fractured
        Cervical third
        Middle third
        Apical third

Class 5   Tooth displaced
        Concussion
        Subluxation
        Dislocation
          Extrusion
          Intrusion
          Labiopalatal displacement
        Avulsion

In addition consider:

Bone
  Alveolar fracture
  Jaw fracture

Soft tissues
  Bruising
  Laceration

General
  Skull
  Body

Treatment philosophy

1. Early examination and assessment.
2. Treat emergency injuries, relieve pain, reassure.
3. Decide if the tooth can be saved long-term.
4. Conserve and support recovery of pulp and periodontal structures.
5. Restore the tooth to good function and appearance as soon as possible.

  Description of treatment can be divided into three time periods:

A. Emergency Treatment
B. Intermediate Treatment
C. Long-term Review

Treatment procedures for permanent teeth

Class 0 – Intact: no fracture, but enamel cracked

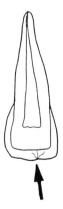

Figure 9.1 Intact enamel

Tooth remains intact and either firm or very slightly loosened in the socket (see Concussion). 'Crazing' of the enamel can be detected upon transillumination of the tooth although there has been no actual tissue loss.

Emergency treatment
This injury is usually ignored by the patient and is only discovered by the dental surgeon at a routine inspection or when a resultant periodontitis or infected necrotic pulp needs treatment.

Consider relieving the bite on the sensitive tooth if it is seen soon after injury.

Intermediate treatment
Review in 7–10 days and repeat pulp tests. Consider fissure sealing the cracked enamel surface.

Long-term review
Pulp vitality tests at regular intervals. The pulp may die and need root canal therapy later. Teeth with open apices at the time of injury are less likely to lose their pulpal vitality.

Class 1 – Enamel fractured

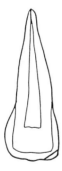

Figure 9.2 Enamel fractured

Emergency treatment
This depends upon the extent of the enamel loss.

1. Leave without treatment.
2. Smooth the sharp edges with sandpaper discs.
3. Acid-etch restoration.

Intermediate treatment
Review the condition in 7–10 days' time and repeat the pulp tests.
In some cases gradual recontouring of the chipped enamel can be
achieved by selective grinding from time to time over a long period
of, say, 12–24 months without the need for restoration at all.

Long-term review
Pulp vitality tests at regular intervals.

Class 2 – Dentine fractured

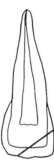

Figure 9.3 Dentine fractured

This injury immediately threatens the vitality of the pulp. Unlike the
slower intrusion of dental caries which gives the tissues time to
react, dentine fracture opens the dentinal tubules to immediate,
direct stimulation from the mouth.

Emergency treatment

1. Isolate the tooth.
2. Estimate how close the fracture is to causing pulpal exposure,
   but do not probe the surface. If the tooth fragment has been
   recovered examine the fractured surface under magnification
   for evidence of pulpal exposure.
3. Seal the dentine surface with calcium hydroxide, the either:
   (a) Cover the calcium hydroxide and the rest of the tooth with
       unfilled clear fissure sealant (e.g. Delton). Allow the first
       layer of sealant to set, wipe it dry and apply a second coat.
   (b) Cover the tooth with a transparent crown form (e.g. Pella)
       filled with temporary cement, or

(c) Restore the tooth by the acid-etch composite technique, improving the retention either by bevelling the enamel margins, preparing a 'mini jacket crown' shoulder preparation or using retention pins. Keep the junction outline between the composite and the sound enamel in a serpentine line that does not attract the eye in the way that a straight line junction does.

Intermediate treatment
Review the condition in 7–10 days' time. Repeat the pulp tests.
    Restore the tooth where this has not already been done.

Long-term review
Repeat the pulp vitality tests at regular intervals. With large acid-etch composite restorations consider the possibility of constructing a porcelain veneer at a later stage to improve the appearance further.

Class 3 – Pulp exposed

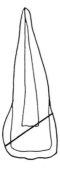

Figure 9.4 Pulp exposed

Treatment will vary depending upon how long the pulp has been exposed to the mouth, the vitality of the pulp, how large the exposure is and whether the apex of the tooth is still open.

Emergency treatment

Pulp capping (see Chapter 6).   Indications: A recent (less than 3 hours), small (less than 2 mm in diameter) exposure in a vital tooth with a good blood supply via an open apex.

Pulpotomy (see Chapter 6).   Indications: A large traumatic exposure, open to the mouth for several hours, with a vital pulp, in a tooth with an open apex.

Apexification (see Chapter 6).   In cases where the pulp, in a tooth with an open apex, has been exposed for a long period or the pulp has become clinically infected the technique of apexification may be attempted.

Pulpectomy.   Where the tooth has a closed apex and the pulp condition has been compromised it may be advisable to commence full root canal therapy and root filling.

Intermediate treatment
Review the tooth in 7–10 days.

Capping: Check the vitality of the tooth.

Pulpotomy: Take radiographs in about 6 weeks and look for signs of the formation of a dentine bridge in the pulp chamber under the capping material.

Root Canal Therapy and Root Filling: Continue in the conventional way.

Long-term review

Capping: Monitor the tooth and pulp vitality at regular intervals.

Pulpotomy: Monitor the tooth radiographically to ensure apical closure occurs.

Apexification: Monitor the tooth radiographically to ensure apical closure occurs and then carry out a conventional root filling.

Crown/root fracture

These fractures extend from the crown to include dental tissues below the level of the gingival attachment. They may occur with or without pulpal involvement. Clinically, in the majority of cases, one part of the crown is mobile while the other section remains firmly attached to the root. Sometimes the injury is more extensive and the tooth is broken into more than two pieces.

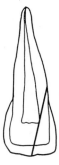

Figure 9.5 Crown/root fracture

Emergency treatment
Under local anaesthesia the mobile fragment of tooth is removed so that the full extent of the injury may be explored. Treatment choices depend upon whether the fracture is simple or multiple and how far the fracture has extended below the gingival level. Where this extension is less than about 4 mm there is a possibility that the tooth may be preserved by gingival contouring and the construction of a crown at a later stage. Where the fracture is multiple or the fracture extends further than 4 mm subgingivally the tooth should be extracted.

If the pulp is exposed a root treatment or pulpotomy should be carried out depending upon the stage of development of the tooth. The gingiva is packed in position with a periodontal pack material and a stainless steel crown fitted.

Intermediate and long-term care
This is devoted to completion of the root canal therapy where the pulp was exposed, monitoring the re-epithelialization of the gingival surface and the construction of a permanent restoration such as a crown constructed on a post and core, a three-quarter crown or a metal/porcelain crown such that the lost subgingival tooth tissue is replaced in gold.

Class 4 – Root fracture

Generally these fractures are curved and circuitous and unless the fragments are displaced they can be difficult to diagnose with certainty. Successful treatment results in healing with a callus of cementum or resorption at the fracture site followed by an ingrowth of bone or connective tissue. Any infection at the fracture site will lead to more extensive tooth resorption and failure to heal.

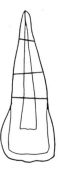

Figure 9.6 Root fractured

Emergency treatment
In general, for both apical and middle third fractures, it is not advisable to extend any endodontic treatment beyond the line of fracture. The coronal fragment should be treated with calcium hydroxide therapy like an immature tooth with an open apex to encourage calcific healing.

Apical third fracture   There is a good chance that the periodontal structure will repair and hold the fragments together firmly over the long term. Splint the tooth for 6 weeks.

Middle third fracture   Perhaps the most difficult to treat. The coronal fragment must be considered to be at least as long below the socket margin level as the crown is above if it is to be firm enough to survive occlusal forces. Splint the tooth for 6 weeks.

Coronal third fracture   Generally the crown of the tooth has been lost and the remaining root should be considered for root canal therapy and the construction of a post and core for a permanent crown.

In cases where the root surface is below the margins of the socket the root may be root filled (perhaps via a tube cemented temporarily into the root canal) and subsequently brought to a more favourable level by orthodontic means before a post and core crown is constructed. Commence root canal therapy or extract.

Teeth with oblique root fractures extending from gingival level to the middle third and beyond, or with multiple root fractures usually require extraction although new techniques are constantly evolving to deal with teeth formerly considered to have a poor prognosis.

Long-term review
The teeth should be monitored clinically and with radiographs at appropriate intervals.

Class 5 – Tooth displaced

Such injury is common in children because of the elastic bone of the young alveolus and the short roots of immature teeth.

Concussion

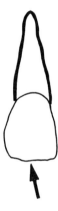

Figure 9.7 Concussion/subluxation

The tooth supporting structures are injured so that the tooth is tender to pressure and percussion, but the tooth is not loose or displaced. The force of the blow has been absorbed by the supporting structures with possible subclinical damage to the periodontal membrane or the apical vessels of a tooth with a closed apex.

Emergency treatment
Relieve the occlusion on the affected tooth by grinding the opposing tooth.

Long-term review
The teeth should be monitored clinically and with vitality tests and radiographs at appropriate intervals.

Subluxation

Like concussion the tooth is tender to pressure and percussion but now is also loose in the socket and there may be some bleeding at the gingival margin.

Treatment: As for concussion.

Dislocation

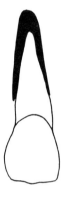

Figure 9.8 Extrusion

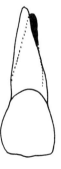

Figure 9.9 Intrusion

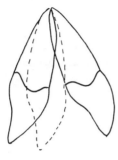

Figure 9.10 Labiopalatal displacement

Extrusion
Intrusion
Labiopalatal displacement

In these instances the displaced tooth has remained in the socket. There is periodontal damage and disruption of the apical tissues, and blood vessels of the tooth in cases of intrusion or lateral displacement the socket walls have been disrupted and there may be an alveolar fracture.

Subluxation, Extrusion, Intrusion, Labiopalatal Displacement:

1. Administer a local anaesthetic.
2. Grasp the tooth with forceps (avoiding the root) or gauze and fingers and move it back into place. In some extrusion cases gentle pressure by the patient from the opposing teeth, steered with a spatula or wooden tongue depressor, can move the tooth into place. Where a tooth has been displaced palatally it may have been forced between momentarily displaced adjacent teeth and not show sufficient room to deliver the crown into place. Try raising such a tooth in the socket until the narrower cervical diameter can allow the tooth to be moved between the adjacent teeth.
3. Splint the tooth.
4. Advise the patient to keep the area clean.
5. Advise a soft diet.

Avulsion ('a tearing apart')

The tooth has been completely dislodged from the socket.

The tooth needs to be replaced urgently if the remaining periodontal tissues on the root are to survive and improve the chances of re-attachment.

Successful replacement depends upon:

1. The length of time the tooth has been out of the mouth; reimplantation after 2 hours has a poor prognosis.
2. The way in which the dislodged tooth has been handled and stored before reimplantation.

Emergency treatment

A. Immediate reimplantation: first aid.

1. Recover the tooth quickly.
2. Handle the tooth with care, trying not to touch the root surface.
3. Clean the root surface by the patient licking it, or by wiping it with a clean handkerchief moistened with the patient's saliva, milk or cold water. *Don't* scrub the tooth or swab it with soap, alcohol or disinfectant.
4. Replace the tooth in the socket, making sure that it is the right way round. (If this can't be done proceed to B.)
5. Get the child to bite on a handkerchief to support the tooth in position.
6. Attend a dental surgery as soon as possible, certainly within 24 hours.

B. Delayed reimplantation: first aid.

If it is impossible to replace the tooth in the socket:

1. Keep the tooth moist:
   (a) In the child's buccal sulcus.
   (b) In the parent's buccal sulcus.
   (c) In a container of milk (an easily obtained physiological solution).
2. Attend a dental surgery immediately, certainly within 2 hours.

C. In the dental surgery.

1. Place the tooth in normal saline.
2. Take a radiograph of the socket and adjacent teeth to check the extent of the injury.
3. Clean the tooth with a saline-moistened gauze and avoid handling the root.

4. Irrigate the socket with saline to remove the blood clot, but do not curette the socket walls.
5. Press the tooth back into place.
6. Splint the tooth in position.
7. Ensure that the child is protected against tetanus or make immediate arrangements in this respect.
8. Decide if antibiotic therapy will be needed.
9. Advise the patient and parent to keep the area clean.
10. Advise soft diet.

Not every avulsed tooth should be reimplanted. If the tooth has already been out of the socket too long to have a good prognosis (95% of teeth reimplanted after more than 2 hours out of the socket are resorbed to some extent later). In some crowded mouths the loss of a unit may be of advantage for future orthodontic treatment plans. However, in most cases reimplantation, even if it fails, is appreciated by the child and parent and gives them time to come to terms with the loss later.

Intermediate care
Review all cases in 7–10 days or see them immediately if the parent or child is at all worried, e.g. the onset of pain or infection.

Dislocation: Cases where the apex of the tooth is open will need careful monitoring and possible calcium hydroxide treatment to encourage apical closure. Teeth with a closed apex generally require root filling.

Extrusion: Leave splinted for 1–2 weeks.

Intrusion or labiopalatal displacement, which includes socket injury: Leave splinted for 3–4 weeks.

Avulsion: Fill the root canal of the reimplanted tooth with calcium hydroxide paste as soon as possible. A necrotic pulp predisposes the complication of external root resorption and ankylosis in re-implanted teeth. Leave the teeth splinted for 1–2 weeks, or if there was a socket injury up to 3–4 weeks. Prolonged rigid splinting reduces the chance of successful periodontal reattachment and may predispose to resorption and ankylosis.

Long-term review
Monitor the injured teeth clinically and radiographically at appropriate intervals.

With displaced teeth be on the look out for root resorption or ankylosis.

Ankylosis occurs where there has been partial root resorption followed by repair by bone or cementum so that the tooth no longer has a periodontal membrane in that region but is united directly to the bone of the alveolus. Clinically ankylosis can be detected by a sound of a 'nail in a wall' if the tooth is percussed and confirmed on radiographic examination. In the young child an ankylosed tooth, locked in the bone, does not grow down at the same rate as adjacent undamaged teeth and may remain in a poor position for future aesthetic appearance or restoration. Such a tooth cannot be moved orthodontically and must be considered for early extraction.

If the tooth is lost:

1. The space may be maintained by a denture followed by the construction of a bridge when the child is full grown.
2. The space may be encouraged to close by orthodontic means and subsequent acid-etch recontouring or crowning of the remaining teeth will give a good aesthetic result.

Splinting methods

1. Foil

An emergency splint may be made from a metal milk bottle top or a yoghurt top foil, cleaned of coloured paint with a solvent. The foil is moulded over the loose tooth and the adjacent teeth, removed and cut with scissors to a convenient size and shape before being cemented into place with temporary cement.

2. Acid-etch composite

Adjacent teeth are etched labially and palatally at the contact points and attached to each other with buttons of composite material, taking care not to interfere with the occlusion (Figure 9.11). This leaves the gingivae free for cleaning and allows a little physiological movement of the teeth involved.

This method is quick and easy and does not involve any delay for laboratory work to be carried out. An orthodontic 'debonding' bur in a slow handpiece is useful for removing the composite at the end of the splinting period. Problems arise if the material is allowed to flow freely into the interdental space because it is extremely difficult to remove it from this region.

3. Acid-etch composite and bar

Where the teeth are separated the spaces may be bridged with wire (paper clip wire will do) or an orthodontic bracket attached to the mid-line of the labial surfaces of the teeth by acid-etch composite. Where a round wire is used it should be bent into a 'U' shape at the attachment points to resist rotatory movement and failure later (Figure 9.11).

4. Cap splint

An alginate impression is taken (petroleum jelly should be painted on the loose tooth first to avoid removing it in the impression). In the laboratory a vacuum-formed thin plastic splint is constructed and this is cemented over the teeth.

5. Removable splint

From an alginate impression a removable acrylic plate is constructed with clasps and wires to stabilize the loose tooth. The plate is removed to clean the teeth and to check the reattachment of the traumatized tooth.

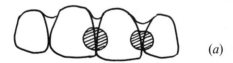

(a)

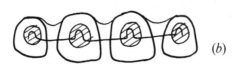

(b)

Figure 9.11 Splint traumatized teeth using (a) acid-etch composite alone, and (b) acid-etch composite and wire where the teeth are widely spaced

Prevention

1. Early orthodontic treatment should be undertaken for children at risk of dental trauma because of protruding teeth.
2. Mouth protectors or mouthguards can be provided which cover the upper teeth and cushion the jaws occlusally. There are several kinds (Welbury and Murray, 1990):
   (a) Ready-made sports shop rubber mouthguards or gum shields in standard small, medium or large sizes. These do not fit very well.
   (b) Mouth-formed polyvinyl plastic (Coe Redigard). These can be adjusted to fit, actually in the athlete's mouth, after they have been softened in hot water for a few moments. Coe also makes a Dental Guard Kit comprising of an outer shell that can be customised by the dentist with a soft acrylic filling layer.
   (c) Specially constructed mouth protectors can be vacuum-formed on a model cast from an alginate impression. In the growing child these appliances must be reviewed at intervals to maintain a good fit as the jaws grow and new teeth erupt.

All mouthguards need to be well washed in cold water after use and stored in a special container. They should be worn during participation in hazardous sports such as boxing, hockey, rugby, football, etc. but unfortunately most accidents occur when the child is unprepared.

Primary teeth

Traumatic injury to the primary teeth presents the operator with less options for treatment than in the permanent dentition. Assessment of the injury must take into account the possibility of a 'knock on' injury to the underlying permanent tooth when a primary tooth is displaced.

Initially the primary tooth roots act as a fence protecting the forming permanent teeth from direct injury. At this stage a vertical blow on the edge of the incisor causes it to slide up over the permanent tooth germ. However, if the crown of the primary tooth is hit from the labial the tooth swings backwards on the fulcrum of the palatal socket margin and this rapid movement of the apex can damage the permanent tooth germ and cause labial enamel hypoplasia.

Later, as the primary incisor gradually resorbs, the effect of trauma can be transmitted to the permanent tooth in different mechanical ways. Finally the stage is reached where the permanent incisor moves forward to lie directly over the resorbed apex of its predecessor (Figure 9.12). Now a vertical blow to the primary tooth is transmitted in such a way that the forming permanent tooth root is disrupted and this can cause dilaceration and other malformations.

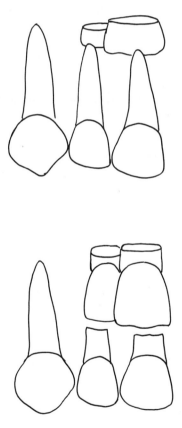

Figure 9.12 Stages of tooth development in the incisal region at age 3 and 5 years to illustrate how trauma to the primary teeth may be transmitted to the forming permanent teeth

Treatment procedures for primary teeth

Intact: No fracture but enamel cracked. Treat as concussion.

All traumatized primary teeth should be kept under regular observation and monitored for any colour change, tenderness or apical sinus, etc. that would indicate pulpal pathology.

Assessment of tooth discoloration following injury to these teeth is an inexact science, but the following interpretations are suggested:

1. Early bruising: haemoglobin from damaged blood vessels in the pulp causing discoloration of the dentine. The tooth may gradually improve in colour like a skin bruise, but the pulp may die.
2. Calcification: yellowish opaque coloration occurring after an interval as the pulp chamber is obliterated.
3. Necrosis: blue colour, can indicate pulpal necrosis. Check apical condition radiographically and consider extraction.

Primary enamel fractured
Sharp edges of enamel should be smoothed or the tooth restored. Keep the tooth under regular observation.

Primary dentine fractured
Restore the tooth and keep it under regular observation.

Primary pulp exposed
Consider pulpotomy and restoration, or extraction.

Primary crown/root fracture
Extract.

Primary root fractured
Remove the coronal fragment but do not attempt to remove the root fragment unless it is loose and easily visible.

Primary tooth displaced
Concussion or Subluxation.
No treatment. Monitor clinically and radiographically as appropriate.

Dislocation

Extrusion and lateral displacement: Under local anaesthesia gently move the tooth back into position with finger pressure. Make sure that there is no danger of the child swallowing or inhaling a very loose tooth; if there is such a danger, extract the tooth. Advise a soft diet and to keep the area clean. Review in 48 hours and at regular intervals subsequently.

Intrusion: Providing that the tooth is firm and not affecting the occlusion, leave the tooth to re-erupt. Moving the intruded tooth may cause damage to the permanent successor. Review the condition in 7–10 days.

Avulsion: Reimplantation of avulsed primary teeth is not advisable because of the risk of damage and infection to the permanent successor.

Chapter 10

Non-accidental injury: child abuse

It is an unpleasant but well documented fact that some children are deliberately injured, abused or neglected by adults, usually their parents. Such injuries can present in many forms but are commonly the result of blows with the hands or fists, or roughly shaking the child.

The condition of non-accidental injury (NAI) is generally progressive in each case and thus, in time, the extent of the injuries gets more and more serious. NAI will occasionally be suspected in children attending for dental treatment, for about 65% of the injuries involve the head and neck. The problem is commonest in children under the age of 3 years and the number of cases is said to be rising. Some 70–80 children die each year in the UK from this kind of abuse.

The dental surgeon has a professional responsibility to be alert to detect these occurrences and to take appropriate action to inform the caring authorities in order to protect the child in future.

Predisposing factors

1. Antisocial, aggressive parent.
2. Bad living conditions and poverty.
3. Frustration caused by family problems, work or mental stress.
4. Very young mothers, perhaps single parent, unwanted pregnancy.
5. Parents with a low baby-crying tolerance.
6. Where child is unwanted and neglected by the rest of the family.

Suspicion

Diagnosis of child abuse, either physical or mental, is often missed. Suspicion should arise in the following circumstances:

1. Inexplicable delay between injury and seeking professional attention.
2. Child brought to an unknown dentist.
3. Accompanying adult is not the parent.
4. Unusual response to the injury by the parent; disturbed reaction. Parent may give either an inadequate or over-plausible and embroidered explanation of how the injury occurred. May exhibit unnatural lack of concern or conversely over-attendance and over-anxiety. There may be attempts to impede a full examination.
5. Child is unnaturally still and alert. May be unwilling to talk.
6. Child shows signs of general neglect.
7. Evidence of repeated injury.
8. History of previous injury to child and siblings.

Types of injury

(Approximately 50% include orofacial injury)
Evidence of blows to the face and neck: facial bruising, finger bruises on the prominent bones of the face.
Damage to the lips, torn fraenum.
Broken or loosened teeth.
Black eye, eye haemorrhage.
Hair pulled out, ears twisted and bruised.
Bite marks.
Scalp bruises.
Skull or jaw fractures.
Cigarette burns or scalds.
Minor bruises where the child has been gripped tightly and shaken.
Complex patterns of skin erythema where child has been beaten with such things as coat hanger, belt buckle, etc.
Fractured bones, limbs, ribs, ruptured internal organs.
Abuse can also be sexual, emotional or due to general neglect with regard to the provision of food, protection, warmth, affection, medical and dental care and in leaving the child unattended.

Management of a suspicious case

1. Be alert.
2. Never make accusations. It is most important to maintain a tactful, courteous demeanour at all times while dealing with every aspect of a suspicious situation.

3. Take a detailed history with adequate records and radiographs and possibly photographs.
4. Check the history from the child separately from the parent if possible.
5. Carry out emergency treatment. In group or hospital practice discuss the case, in confidence, with a colleague.
6. Where necessary refer the child to hospital and telephone to speak to the consultant. Send any letter by post in case it goes astray. Check later that they have kept the appointment.
7. Liaise with local authorities by contacting the child's general practitioner or a member of the Social Services Department or the District Community Physician (both listed in the telephone directory), in confidence. They will be able to check if the child is already on the local register of children 'at risk' and take any necessary action to investigate and protect the child.
8. The dental surgeon should keep an accurate record of who he contacted and when.

In extreme cases of injury a hospital can admit a child and the paediatrician may call upon a magistrate to give authority for the child to be taken into care in a place of safety. This gives the Social Services Department time to take appropriate action for the future.

They have to be aware that taking a child from the family may prove to be destructive in some cases. After careful investigation of the facts alternatives may be found such as gaining help and care from the extended family or by constructively helping the parent through their crisis stage.

All of this unhappy procedure seems far from the normal events of a busy dental practice. However, every professional person who suspects that a child is being abused or neglected has a legal as well as a moral obligation to take the necessary steps to initiate appropriate action.

Chapter 11

Emergencies

Accident prevention

Always protect every child visiting the practice by making sure
that you provide as safe an environment as possible. Pay special
attention to such things as electrical equipment, sockets, trailing
flexes, fires, etc. Look out for items that can be pulled on top of the
child, or fallen over, or picked up and swallowed and so on. Make
sure there are no open windows to fall out of. The list can be
unending but these few examples indicate a basic philosophy of
general vigilance and care.

Remember that to a normally inquisitive child your dental
surgery is an adventure playground filled with numerous fascinating
things such as switches, drawers, sharp instruments and flames,
bottles and boxes. Although the dentist's attention is focused on the
provision of dental care, the child's well-being must be protected as
well. Never leave any child alone and unsupervised in your dental
surgery for he may hurt himself.

In the surgery

Never operate without another person present, preferably a trained
Dental Surgery Assistant.

Make sure that the visiting patient's medical and drug history
is completely up to date so that treatment won't cause drug
reactions, etc.

Watch out for the child who is unwell (trauma, fever, infection,
drug reaction) and be prepared to deal with those whose medical
history predisposes them to some kind of an attack in the surgery.

The dentist is not a complete paediatrician, but he and his staff
must be alert and ready to take primary care in the event of an
emergency. Hold practice sessions of what to do in an emergency.
Keep resuscitation equipment up to date and instantly available
within arm's reach.

Special things about the child

1. While the child is growing and changing it does not have the mature organ systems of an adult and they may react unpredictably in an emergency.
2. A child is not able to withstand profound changes in the fluid balances in the way that an adult can in the event of severe haemorrhage or dehydration (as in severe fever or vomiting).
3. A child's larynx and airway is much smaller than an adult's and is thus more easily obstructed. The trachea size can be estimated as being of about the same diameter as the child's little finger. Any tracheal oedema soon causes respiratory distress. At less than six months the baby is an obligate nose breather.
4. A child's lung capacity is smaller than the adult and any congestion soon causes interruption of the oxygen/carbon dioxide exchange and respiratory distress.

Ambulance

An ambulance will be needed in the following circumstances:

1. Serious outdoor accident.
2. Difficulty in breathing.
3. Heart failure.
4. Severe bleeding.
5. Unconsciousness.
6. Severe burns.
7. Suspected fracture.
8. Shock.
9. Poisoning.

Action

Dial 999.
Ask for the ambulance emergency service.
Give your phone number in case you are cut off.
Give exact location of the incident (plus landmarks to help the driver find it quickly).
What has happened.
Number injured.
Ages of injured.
Extent of injuries.

Don't hang up until told to do so, i.e. before the ambulance control officer does so. Return to incident to confirm to others that the ambulance call has been made.

Bruises

Are common in childhood. Treat with cold water compresses at the time of injury, to limit the extent of the bruise.

Black eye needs careful examination as it may indicate a bony injury of the orbit.

Burns and scalds

1. Immerse the burn in cold water—in a bowl under a running cold water tap. This cools the lesion and soothes the pain.
2. Loosen and remove anything tight that might impede swelling—rings, watches, belts, etc., but don't pull off burnt clothing stuck to the burn.
3. Cover the burn with a wet, clean material and seek urgent medical attention.
4. For serious, extensive burns call an ambulance.

Cardiopulmonary resuscitation

A B C   (Airway, Breathing, Circulation)

Action

A. Airway

1. Lay the child flat.
2. Clear the mouth of any foreign matter.
3. Lift the chin to bring the mandible forward and open the airway.
4. Look and listen for breathing.

B. Breathing

1. If *not* breathing after airway opened,
2. Begin mouth-to-mouth or mouth-to-nose resuscitation. Place your mouth over the child's. Maintain airway position of mandible.

3. Blow gently. For a small child use cheek breathing only. Remember the child's smaller lung capacity. Watch the chest rising. Don't over inflate. For a child of 5–7 years watch out for loose teeth.
4. Allow the air to come out again.
5. Repeat two or three times, then check the circulation.

C. Circulation

1. Feel pulse: inside the upper arm, in the neck, in the chest.
2. If there is a pulse go back to breathing.
3. If there is no pulse go on to heart compression.
4. Place the child on his back on a firm surface or the floor.
5. Find the point a finger breadth above the bottom edge of the child's sternum. Press that point with two fingers compressing the chest some 1–2 cm only, allow the rebound and repeat about once a second.
6. Give five compressions to one breath.
7. If there is assistance alternate the actions, one person taking care of the breathing while the other continues the cardiac compression.

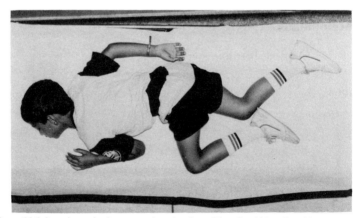

Figure 11.1 A patient who is unconscious but breathing should be placed in the *recovery position*: stomach down, head to one side, the limbs on that side bent with the thigh at right angles to the body and the hand at face level, the other arm behind the body to stabilize it. No pillow should be used under the head. The head must be extended with the chin well forward to open and maintain the airway, and any debris, vomit or blood must be removed from the mouth. The condition of the patient must be monitored constantly

8. Call for medical assistance or an ambulance.
9. If the child begins to recover administer oxygen and nurse him in the recovery position (Figure 11.1) until the ambulance arrives. He must be admitted to hospital for full investigation of the effects of the collapse.

Note: Facial injury may prevent the preferred mouth-to-mouth resuscitation without an airway accessory. In such a case use the Holger–Neilsen technique to ventilate the lungs. Here the patient is placed face down on the floor, head on one side with the cheek supported on the backs of the hands, and with the arms raised as high as possible. Then, with the operator kneeling at the casualty's head some respiratory exchange can be gained by alternately compressing the rib cage and raising the elbows. This brief description is intended as a reminder and is not sufficient to allow the reader to carry out this technique properly. The precise details of this method should be learned from a standard First Aid text (e.g. British Red Cross).

Choking/respiratory obstruction

Predisposing factors

1. Food. Infants and toddlers can choke on food and solids that are not properly chewed up. They should not be given peanuts, chunky viscous foods or sweets.
2. Medicines. Pills or tablets should never be prescribed for babies and toddlers but replaced by drops or elixirs.
3. Foreign bodies. Infants like exploring things with the mouth. Small items can get swallowed. In the dental surgery a child might accidentally swallow such things as a dental bur or an extracted tooth. If a dental object is lost, inhaled or swallowed, even if it appears to be symptomless, inform the parent and make sure that the child is immediately referred to hospital for appropriate investigation and treatment. This may include radiographic examination of the chest and abdomen followed by bronchoscopy or cotton wool sandwiches and monitoring of the faeces until the item is recovered. Sharp or toxic items require immediate care at a hospital Accident and Emergency Department.

Action for a conscious, choking child

1. Check if the child can breathe easily and cough up the item.

2. Ask 'Are you choking?' and if they cannot reply proceed to invert the child over your knee, head down and bang him on the back between the shoulder blades.
3. Turn the toddler on his back, well supported, e.g. on your lap or on the ground, and perform 4–5 chest thrusts pushing on the lower sternum with two or three fingers only. For a bigger child, put him on his back on the ground, kneel at his feet, place one hand on the upper abdominal area away from the xiphoid process of the sternum and execute 6–10 firm upward abdominal thrusts. These gentler modifications of the Heimlich manoeuvre cause sudden increases of intrapulmonary pressure that can expel a foreign body from the throat.
4. Check in the mouth again and remove the obstruction if you can.
5. If there is still no improvement and the child loses consciousness call for help and start full cardiopulmonary resuscitation procedures (see above).

Drug reaction/anaphylaxis

This is caused by a drug allergy, e.g. sensitivity to penicillin. It will occur more frequently in patients with a history of other allergies, asthma, eczema or hay fever.

Within half an hour after being given the drug in question the patient feels cold in the extremities, uneasy and agitated, and begins to wheeze with a bronchospasm. They develop an urticarious itchy rash, angioedema of the face and eyelids. In severe cases there is sudden hypotension and circulatory collapse with loss of consciousness, cold clammy skin and a weak pulse: this patient is in considerable danger.

Action

Place the patient flat on his back and raise his legs to maintain the circulation to the higher centres in the brain.

Administer
Adult dose (BNF): 1 ml of 1/1000 adrenaline which contains adrenaline 1 mg/ml, given by intramuscular injection.
Child dose: 10 μg/kg administered slowly over a period of 5 min up to a maximum of 500 μg, given by intramuscular injection.
Give the patient oxygen and summon medical assistance or an ambulance immediately. If there is delayed recovery, the adrenaline

injection should be repeated after 15 min. In severely affected patients medical treatment may include hydrocortisone sodium succinate (Dose: 1–5 years 50 mg; 6–12 years 100 mg; adult 200 mg) injected slowly into a vein. The patient should be kept under observation in hospital for 24 hours to check for complications and in case of a relapse. Afterwards they must carry a card warning them and others of their drug allergy.

Epileptic fit

Grand mal. The child will have a warning aura and give a cry before becoming rigid and losing consciousness followed by jerking movements of the limbs and frothing at the mouth.

Action

Keep calm. The fit must run its course without interference. Move the child to a clear space, so that he won't hurt himself, and if possible put a pad under his head. Loosen any tight clothing around the neck. Don't put anything into the child's mouth. An epileptic fit is self-limiting and only if it lasts for more than 10 min should it require medical assistance. When the seizure is over, nurse the child in the recovery position and make sure that he has fully recovered before allowing him to go home.

Fainting

May be caused by physical or emotional stimuli such as pain, fear, an over-heated room, the sight of blood, etc. The child feels light-headed and dizzy, turns very pale and may lose consciousness with a slow, weak pulse and shallow breathing. The condition improves quickly if the patient is placed on his back in a horizontal position with the feet raised, and any tight clothing around the neck, chest and waist loosened. After recovery he should not be allowed to stand up again too quickly.

Poisoning

Prevention

1. Make sure drugs are dispensed in a child-proof container. Never actually hand a child a supply of drugs, or such things as

fluoride tablets or mouthwash. *Always* hand to the responsible adult.
2. Make sure that the responsible adult understands how important it is to keep drugs out of the reach of children and to supervise their use.

Note on the acute toxicity of fluoride: Smith *et al.* (1986) report that the lethal toxic dose of fluoride is now considered to be 14–28 mg/kg bodyweight. They calculate that this means that if a 5-year-old child weighing 20 kg swallows two-thirds of a 500 ml bottle of 0.2% sodium fluoride rinse, this could be lethal. Furthermore, only 32 ml of a 2% solution could be lethal and 2.2 ml would be enough to cause acute symptoms. These cautions are echoed by other authorities.

Action

Stay calm.

1. Try to identify the agent and the amount taken and when.
2. If possible try to empty the stomach. This must not be attempted if the child has swallowed a corrosive or is actually unconscious. Vomiting can be induced after the child has taken a drink of water or milk by stimulating the back of the throat with a spoon handle. A doctor might consider giving an emetic containing Ipecacuanha.
3. If a fluoride overdose has been taken give the child plenty of milk to drink for it will tend to fix the fluoride. Even though there may be no symptoms in this case further hospital treatment is urgent.
4. In all cases refer the child to hospital urgently for further assessment, and possible antidote therapy, gastric lavage, and supportive treatment.

Reference

Smith, B. G. N., Wright, P. S. and Brown, D. (1986) The clinical handling of dental materials. Wright, Bristol

Chapter 12

Handicapped children

A handicapped child is defined as one who, over an appreciable period of time, is prevented from full participation in childhood activities of a social, recreational, educational and vocational nature (World Health Organization). The term 'disabled' is often preferred; thus a disabled child in a wheelchair is handicapped by the environment when he has to negotiate stairs.

Classification

Handicaps may be classified as mental, physical, emotional, medical or, for completeness, social.

The problems range from those of children with something organically wrong but who are not in an accepted sense ill (e.g. deafness, cerebral palsy or mental handicap) to children who suffer chronic disease lasting for long periods and with life-long effects (e.g. asthma, cystic fibrosis and haemophilia). These children with special needs deserve the highest standard of dental care that can be provided for them. To achieve this the dentist must be prepared to adapt and modify his treatment techniques, to gain a wider knowledge of the handicapping condition and to be sensitively aware of its social and emotional effects on the child and its family.

Family

Severe physical or mental handicaps may be apparent at birth, may become manifest later, or be acquired as a result of an accident or severe illness. They will have profound effects on the child's parents and family. At first there will be an element, to a varying extent, of shock, disbelief and denial. This, in the case of the newborn, may be followed by vacillating acceptance or even total rejection. The parents may react to the stress by feeling responsible, ashamed and guilty for the occurrence; they may become angry and seek a scape-goat, or they may even indulge in fantasies about a magic cure.

At the same time, the parents' grief for 'the child that never was' may have serious effects on the siblings and in some cases destroy the family.

Parents may unwittingly, yet understandably, proceed to over-indulge the handicapped child, not coming to terms with the reality, and protecting their 'lame duckling' from outside care agencies. This is counter-productive and damaging for the child's future prospects of using and developing its accessible faculties and potential to the maximum. Early detection and referral for specialist assessment and advice is of prime importance. All child care agencies, including the dentist, must be on the lookout for these problems because some disorders, unlike major malformations, only come to light gradually. For example, a child's hearing and speech should be satisfactory by the age of 5 years or its social and educational adjustments may be marred. However, in the protected home environment such problems can easily remain unnoticed.

Parents faced with the unexpected problems of a child with grave handicaps need counselling and support from the start. They need to be in contact with the Handicap Team usually composed of a paediatrician, general medical practitioner, social workers, psychologist, community nurses, physiotherapist and in some cases the dentist. If the child is well enough to live at home the parents need advice and help about everyday practical management problems. They need support from the Community Services, such as district nurses and social workers, they need to be put in touch with relevant societies and local groups of parents who themselves have suffered the same problem. In some cases parents also need to be given short-term relief from time to time for holidays, days off, weekends, etc. when other caring agencies will look after the handicapped children for them. They will need advice about local special schools.

Public

Public reaction to the appearance and disability of the handicapped child may stigmatize him through curiosity, fear, revulsion or pity. This can affect the child's self-concept and confidence and be very distressing.

The 'handicapped' knows how 'normals' identify him but may still have a sense of not knowing how others really think about him. He may become shy, or attempt a hostile bravado.

Child

The handicapped child's approach to life is complicated both by the disability and the attitude of those caring for him. He may have to endure long periods of sickness and hospitalization. The handicap may block both approaches to him and his own attempts to communicate with the outside world. In general the most important thing is to help him to accept the inevitable and to make the most of what is left.

The chronically sick child

This child has often had to endure prolonged separation from the security of parents and home during periods in hospital. He has had to experience illness, pain, fear and anxiety, distress and possible operations. He may not have understood the need for elective treatment, the operation 'to make you better' when he did not feel too bad anyway. The child's education and play is interrupted. After prolonged periods in hospital this child will have constructed a rapport with the hospital staff and other patients only to find it disrupted when he is discharged to return home again. His life experience has been unusually distorted.

Recent progress

Currently the physically and mentally handicapped are receiving much more attention than they did a generation ago. As a result of this, and the continuing development of medical and surgical skills, an increasing number of these children survive and are able to fit into the community better, for now instead of living in institutions, they can live at home.

Dental care

The trend to make the lives of the handicapped as secure, predictable and normal as possible means that they increasingly seek routine dental care from the general practice.

Dental treatment of children with less severe problems, e.g. deafness, blindness or Down's syndrome is well within the scope of the caring general practitioner and the routine care of these patients within the normal community will be far less upsetting for all concerned. It will be less of an 'occasion' to visit the dentist, and travel, etc. will be less disruptive in the context of a busy and probably uncomfortable life. Nevertheless, in many cases a lot of organization, cost and effort is needed to arrange a visit to the dental surgery, for the child and those taking care of him.

Pre-visit questions

There are several question that need to be answered at the outset when arranging a dental appointment.

What kind of handicap does the child have? Does the child live at home or in an institution? Who is the child's medical adviser? How urgent is the dental treatment needed? Who will give consent for treatment? How will the child travel to the surgery? Public transport? Private car? Ambulance? Who will accompany the child?

Is it necessary to consult the medical adviser first? For example, to learn about the drug history, and if premedication or antibiotic cover needs to be arranged before the child arrives.

The dental practice

Architectural barriers in the physical aspects of the building must be considered. Access to the surgery may require ramps or a lift where the handicap makes it difficult to negotiate stairs. Can the child gain access to the toilet? What about the waiting area, will the child be at ease there? Some of these children may have an unusual appearance or involuntarily make sudden noises which might affect other visitors to the practice.

Staff

The dental surgery assistant must be specially trained and rehearsed to work with these cases, and to cope with the child's special needs.

Equipment

Most of these special patients can be treated in the normal dental surgery, but certain aspects of flexibility will allow the room to be adapted to a particular child's needs. A spacious surgery gives the physically handicapped more room to manoeuvre without knocking into things. It will help if the main surgery equipment can be repositioned to allow treatment to be carried out for patients confined to a wheelchair.

Treatment can be facilitated in some cases by the use of various mouth props, finger guards and other small items which the dentist tends to choose for himself. Some patients can be supported, stabilized and made more comfortable in the dental chair with pillows, bean bags and small sandbags, or by being wrapped in a sheet.

Make sure that the surgery and waiting area can be cleaned up easily in event of any spillages, etc.

General treatment philosophy

1. Assessment
2. Prevention
3. Operative treatment
4. Maintenance.

Most of these children react to dentistry in a similar way to the normal child and are fearful, appreciative and cooperative within the bounds of their mental or physical condition. Treatment to a high standard demands many changes in thinking and techniques of dental treatment as well as an understanding of the handicapping condition.

An understanding and caring attitude can go a long way in coping with the routines of dental care in these cases.

The first stage is to make an assessment of dental needs. Then attention must be directed to encouraging prevention: dietary advice, the use of fluorides, attention to improving and maintaining oral hygiene as much as possible (for it can be very difficult in some cases), consider the use of plaque-reducing mouthwashes (Corsodyl), and the need for frequent monitoring dental inspections.

Restorative treatment should be carried out to the highest standard possible. Treatment may be attempted by conventional means, but sometimes the severity of the handicap or the urgency of a neglected mouth may require that dental treatment is undertaken under a general anaesthetic, preferably in a specialized centre associated with a hospital. Many of these cases can be treated on a day-stay basis with competent anaesthetist and good nursing care. They will probably be less upset if they can return to their own bed to sleep that night and certainly less upset and disruptive than if they have to spend the night or two in a general ward unable to understand or come to terms with the strange surroundings.

Once the mouth has been set right it is then good policy to maintain the condition by regular follow-up care, in many cases assisted by a dedicated oral hygienist.

In general, it must be remembered that most of these children have a whole life span ahead of them and that they deserve the very best dental care that can be provided for them in order that a dental problem does not further affect their already reduced life style.

Not every dentist is emotionally equipped to deal with the very worst handicaps of some of these children. If the dentist cannot maintain a professional attitude to these patients he should not force himself to try. The added load upon him, in addition to the professional load and requirement, becomes too great. Nevertheless he has a duty to ensure that the child receives the best of dental care by making the necessary referral to a specialist at an early stage.

Domiciliary visits

Some handicapped children will require treatment at home. Portable equipment is now available to bring light, a dental engine and suction to the armchair or bedside. The operator and his assistant need to practice with this equipment before attempting to use it in strange surroundings. They must also rehearse which instruments, drugs and materials will be required as well. It is important to update the medical history before making the visit and to have all the lines of communication and help adequately arranged in the event of an emergency.

After-care should be explained carefully and written down as well so that there are no mistakes afterwards. This is a good opportunity to update advice about preventive dentistry: diet, oral hygiene and fluorides.

Examples of treatment strategies

Blind or partially sighted

These start their training before the age of two. Education is usually given in a residential school.

The blind or partially sighted person must be guided while they are moving about in the unfamiliar dental surgery environment, particularly with regard to things they can trip over or bump into. The dentist should concentrate on the good channels of communication: sound and touch, He must try to convey, in what he says and in the tone of his voice, his concern for the patient's well-being, his 'time to listen' and 'time to explain'. He should try to build up routines that will make the child feel safe, starting with where to put their coat each time they come to visit the surgery. The child is led to the dental chair and allowed to feel the surfaces before climbing into it. Every new thing should be explained immediately, repeatedly if necessary, e.g. when adjusting the chair. Also when the dentist touches the patient's face and mouth, he should warn them beforehand and do it gently and explain the sounds and sensations of what he is doing.

The dentist can keep up a running commentary but must also allow the child to ask all the questions he needs to, for thus he is able to explore a new person and get to know them. He may want to feel the instrument with his fingers before it is used. This can be allowed if the instrument is not sharp but it may mean that a new sterile one is needed for the treatment. Some children may be allowed to have a hand on the dentist's while he carries out treatment procedures. Blind patients still need eye protection when lying back in the chair.

Deaf

The deaf or partially hearing child needs to be discovered and taught early or they may remain dumb. These children usually attend residential schools until they can lipread well enough to attempt integration into normal school.

The condition may be discovered when it is noticed that the child does not attempt to listen and does not respond to his name and, by the age of three, may also have delayed speech. Various hearing tests are available from a very early age but by the age of 4 years such a child must have had a specialist examination and audiometry tests if its potential for learning speech is to be rescued. Some children may have to be given a hearing aid. This not only helps to amplify the sounds of speech but also serves to identify the problem to a stranger like a blind person's white stick. However, even the best hearing aid cannot filter the sound input and there are problems of distortion and the pick-up of extraneous sound. Although complete deafness is rare, in some cases the child may never have heard speech properly, others may have lost part of the whole spectrum of sound at a later date and thus have learned the value of words and then been deprived of the facility to hear them clearly.

Faced with these children the dentist is soon made aware that he cannot use one of his most important channels of communication and reassurance: the soothing voice, soft tone, the verbal explanation of treatment.

Where the child has partial hearing it is best to speak in a normal clear voice; not to shout and not to space out and emphasize words. A lot of the meaning of speech is transferred by the inflection of the voice and the rhythm of the sentence, even when the words are blurred by a narrowed spectrum of sound appreciation. The speaker should try to keep the sentences short and sharp and be aware of the difficulty of communicating verb tenses. Confusing background noise must be kept to a minimum. In many cases the child may have learned to lipread, or has a parent or friend who can interpret between the dentist and the patient by finger spelling.

When communicating with a deaf person the dentist should arrange to stand squarely in front of them and make sure that his face is in a good light. This gives them a chance to see his facial expression, eye contact and non-verbal gestures and to gain re-assurance about him before he places them in the supine position and sits behind them. Necessary eye protection should be provided but with clear glasses so that they can still see. The deaf child may be bothered by the unusual vibrations caused by dental treatment; a hearing aid may be affected by the noise and even with the aid switched off, some deaf patients are aware of the sounds of dental treatment on their teeth because of bone conduction.

Wheelchair cases

The child in a wheelchair may present problems with regard to transport to the surgery. They usually have to travel by car or ambulance and with someone to help them to negotiate problems of the terrain. Cars entitled to a special 'disabled' badge are allowed special dispensations over any restrictions for car parking near to the practice.

The practice needs to have wide doors, ramps not stairs, or a lift. In the surgery there may not be any need to move the child from the wheelchair to the dental chair if the bracket table, operating light, unit etc. can be easily regrouped.

The wheelchair should have its brakes on. The child's head has to be supported during treatment. This can be achieved by putting the chair against a wall, with or without a cushion, or by having someone support the head from behind, or better still, by having a special headrest that can be temporarily attached to the wheelchair itself.

Otherwise the child has to be lifted into the dental chair and adequately supported by pillows, sand-bags etc. using the chair's flexibility to achieve an acceptable compromise between the patient and the operator's needs for a comfortable operating position.

Mental handicap

Some mentally handicapped children may have normal bodies but many suffer multiple handicaps with problems of physical development, heart defects, impaired hearing and sight, etc. The handicap may be due to brain damage at birth, meningitis or injury.

Mongolism or Down's syndrome is associated with chromosomal abnormality (trisomy 21). Nearly half of these children have heart lesions such as a ventriculoseptal defect (VSD).

Cases of mental deficiency may be classified according to the results of a test to find the Intelligence Quotient (IQ) which relates the 'mental age' to the chronological age.

90–120	Normal
50–70	ESN(M) moderately educationally subnormal
0–50	ESN(S) severely educationally subnormal

The results of such tests have to be interpreted carefully for they are affected by experience and learning. These children also need to be studied over a period of time in an assessment centre.

In the dental surgery a wide spectrum of cooperation can be expected, from docile acceptance through retarded understanding to aggressive resistance. Down's syndrome children are friendly, affectionate and usually easy to manage.

Initial management problems include difficulties of communication and language interpretation of meaning by the patient, who may also have a short attention span and a poor memory. The dentist should try not to confuse the patient by introducing too many new stimuli, and at all times try to develop a feeling of security and confidence.

It is important to allow plenty of time to consider the patient's condition, the full medical history, and to gain a full understanding of the problem. The dentist should try to discover the ways in which the parents and others may be able to control behaviour. It is also important to allow the child sufficient time to come to terms with the new and frightening surroundings. Many of these children will begin to respond to the dentist as they gain confidence in each other so that routine dental care can proceed.

At the other extreme, problems in the chair can include total lack of cooperation, hitting out at instruments, biting the dentist and his staff, closing heavily on instruments such as mouth mirrors and breaking them. There may be sudden uncontrolled movements of the head so that excavators or engines can get caught in the soft tissues. Further difficulties may include the child shouting, crying and even losing control of its bladder and bowels (a good reason for getting the patient to visit the toilet before coming into the surgery).

Sudden loud screams can be disconcerting for the operator and staff and particularly for patients in the waiting room unless you have arranged for them to be given prior warning that it might happen. In such cases treatment has to be carried out under general anaesthesia.

Although most of these children live at home some may be institutionalized and thus potential carriers of blood-borne diseases such as hepatitis.

Infantile autism (Kanner's syndrome)

In this condition there is a profound impairment of the child's ability to relate to people. The cause is unknown, but it may be due to brain injury or constitutional vulnerability. There is delayed speech, and social smiling is also delayed or absent. The infant is not 'cuddly' and never reaches up to be picked up. There is minimal eye contact. The child remains withdrawn and solitary preferring toys, activities and rituals to parents and people, becoming angry if a ritual is disturbed. There is a tendency to become obsessed with trivia, e.g. always insisting on drinking from the same coloured cup. Intelligence ranges from normal to severely subnormal. The initial poor language skill and understanding tends to persist and the child may repeat back what is said to it often using 'you' for 'I'. In some cases the child may become aggressive, self-mutilating, hyperactive and antisocial.

Treatment strategies include antipsychotic drug therapy and attendance at a therapeutic residential school.

In the dental surgery the operator must have patience and be prepared for the unpredictable.

Cerebral palsy

This is the general term used to describe a group of non-progressive motor disorders arising from intrauterine, perinatal or accidental damage to the central nervous system and characterized by varying degrees of impaired muscular functions and voluntary movement. The problems may be classified as spastic, athetoid or ataxic.

Spastic: The limbs may be affected to a varying degree and the condition may be hemiplegic, paraplegic or quadraplegic. In the latter case the mouth, tongue and palate movement are commonly affected and there are difficulties with swallowing, feeding, speaking and dribbling. The limbs affected are 'floppy' or subject to spasms and there is difficulty in walking, sitting and hand movement.

Athetoid: Writhing involuntary movement with abrupt jerky movement that increase with nervousness or emotional tension and disappears during sleep.

Ataxic: Less common. Weak, uncoordinated, unsteady with an intention tremor that upsets rapid or fine movements.

Associated disorders include convulsions, eye defects, hearing defects.

Many spastic children have normal intelligence although some are mentally retarded.

Dental problems include:

1. Malocclusion due to muscle imbalances.
2. Enamel defects due to intrauterine environment.
3. Gingival problems with anti-epilepsy drugs.
4. Physical difficulties in maintaining oral health.

Treatment problems arise because of difficulties with communication between the operator and patient and in keeping the child still in the chair. A small child may be supported and its uncontrolled movements restrained on the parent's knee, while an older one may be restrained in a variety of ways with sand bags, seat belt straps, velcro straps, wrapping up in a sheet, etc. The mouth may be held open during treatment by the use of rubber mouth props, gags, the handle of a toothbrush, wooden tongue depressors taped together or metal finger guards. In every case it must be explained to the patient that the restraint is used to help them to cooperate more easily, not as a means of force.

Heart disease

This term is used to describe a wide range of heart conditions which are mostly congenital structural defects of heart muscle or valves and the associated great vessels, but may be acquired as the result of infection such as rheumatic fever. The resultant cardiac insufficiency makes the child short of breath, easily fatigued and even cyanosed. The presence of a heart murmur may be one sign of heart disease, although many such murmurs may be found to be insignificant by the cardiologist. Congenital deformities may improve spontaneously with age or need to be treated by operation.

Medical advice should be sought before attempting dental treatment for such children with regard to fitness for anaesthesia and the necessity for antibiotic prophylaxis of infective endocarditis before dental treatment. In most at-risk cases the child carries a card from the cardiologist describing the antibiotic regimen to be followed. Local anaesthetics containing adrenaline should be avoided for patients with unstable cardiac rhythms. In case of accidental intravenous injection. prilocaine with or without felypressin has been suggested (BNF). Preventive care should be initiated to reduce the need for operative dental treatment in the future.

Infective bacterial endocarditis

Children with cardiac defects (rheumatic fever history, valve lesions, 'hole in the heart', cardiac surgery, etc.) must be considered to be at risk of developing infective bacterial endocarditis following any dental treatment which may cause transient bacteraemia, e.g. dental extractions, scaling, periodontal surgery, etc. Some authorities include all dental treatment in this list. Any child at risk must be given antibiotic cover before dental treatment. Children who have already had infective endocarditis before should be referred to hospital for dental treatment.

Most special risk patients carry a card outlining the precise antibiotic regimen to be given before dental treatment, otherwise advice should be sought from the child's GP or specialist. Always report any adverse after-effects to the child's medical adviser.

Currently, guidelines for antibiotic cover are suggested as follows:

1. Child not sensitive to penicillin. Oral amoxycillin given one hour before the dental operation (Adult dose: 3 g; Child: under 5, quarter adult dose; 5–10, half adult dose; over 10, adult dose. BNF). This prophylaxis may be safely repeated after an interval of a month if further treatment is required. When a general anaesthetic is necessary and the patient has to be starved preoperatively, amoxycillin may be given four hours prior to induction, with the administration of a further dose immediately upon recovery.
2. Child sensitive to penicillin. Oral erythromycin stearate given one hour before the dental operation and a second dose 6 hours later (Adult dose: 1.5 g; Child: under 5, quarter adult dose; 5–10, half adult dose; over 10, adult dose. BNF). When a general anaesthetic is necessary the child should be referred to hospital.
3. If neither drug is appropriate (e.g. erythromycin stearate may cause nausea and vomiting in some cases), contact the child's doctor or specialist for advice.
4. In all cases the antibiotic premedication must be actually taken in the presence of the dental surgeon or a delegated member of his staff.

Bleeding disorders

A variety of bleeding disorders occur, generally inherited, mainly the haemophilias or von Willebrand disease which are caused by deficiency of Factor VIII in the blood clotting mechanism. In suspected cases check the history, for most affected children have suffered some bleeding crisis at an early age such as haemarthrosis, haematoma, prolonged bleeding after dental extraction or tonsillectomy. Diagnostic screening is by blood count, bleeding and clotting time and prothrombin time.

Bleeding episodes at home can now be family-treated by the use of cryoprecipitates. Human Factor VIII should be administered to produce effective levels before any surgery.

Sickle-cell disease

The term used for a group of disorders of haemoglobin formation. The most serious of these is sickle-cell anaemia: so-called because the red blood cells become sickle-shaped when they give up oxygen. The condition is inherited from parents who themselves are carriers of the sickle-cell trait. The disorder is found commonly in black people of African or Caribbean descent. Approximately 1 in 10 has the trait and 1 in 400 has sickle-cell anaemia. It can also occur in people from the East Mediterranean, Middle East, India and Pakistan. An early screening for the presence of sickle-cell anaemia is important for those children at risk. An affected child is likely to suffer from a crisis in conditions which cause a reduced level of oxygen in the blood such as infections, high fever, dehydration, or certain general anaesthetic procedures; sickling of the red blood cells with occlusion of blood vessels may occur. No child from the groups known to be at risk should be given a general anaesthetic without first discovering the result of a screening test. If the disorder is present the child will require the care of a specialist anaesthetist in hospital. Screening is carried out initially by a simple sickle-cell test (Sickledex) on a small blood sample. If the test is positive a further laboratory haemoglobin electrophoresis examination is required to differentiate between trait and anaemia.

Malignancies

These fall into two categories in children: those arising from developing tissue such as neuroblastomas (from the neural crest and sympathetic ganglia), nephroblastomas (from the kidney) and retinoblastomas (from the eye); and those found at all ages.

Intensive treatment by chemotherapy or radiotherapy at a paediatric oncology centre puts a considerable strain on the child and its family who need support and understanding. Any dental procedures carried out during the treatment and recovery period will generally be of an emergency nature because of toothache and must be done in close cooperation with the paediatrician in charge. Every effort should be made to work without tiring or distressing the child. Ideally all potential extractions, root canal therapy or dental infections should have been dealt with before the commencement of radiotherapy in the region of the mouth, because of the danger of radionecrosis.

One side-effect of radiotherapy or chemotherapy will be the interruption of normal growth of the dental structures. A high proportion of dental anomalies can occur subsequently such as hypodontia, microdontia, enamel hypoplasia and abnormal root structure. In some cases there is delayed tooth eruption (Maguire *et al.*, 1987).

Cleft lip and palate

Team work: Plastic surgeon, paediatrician, orthodontist, paedodontist, oral hygienist, speech therapist, district nurse all work together.

Initial problems include the need for construction of special intraoral appliances to enable the baby to suck and to feed.

Asthma

During an attack this child has problems actually breathing out due to bronchial constriction which prevents air from being driven out of the lung before the next breath is taken in.

An attack may be brought on by exposure to an allergic agent, by stress or in some cases by the child who is seeking the benefits of special care and attention.

The condition generally responds to the use of an inhaler which provides a bronchodilating agent.

The dentist should consult the patient's medical adviser before arranging treatment to discover the known precipitating factors and for advice about general care and precautions in the dental surgery.

The child should bring his inhaler to the surgery. Any dental care must be kept as stress-free as possible.

Cystic fibrosis

Affects the lungs and digestive system. There is a physical change in the exudates from the bronchi and an increased vulnerability to chest infections. These children spend regular periods each day undergoing physiotherapy to clear the chest.

They are not good prospects for general anaesthesia or relative analgesia and frequently require antibiotics to combat infections.

Epilepsy

Maintain oral hygiene because the drugs taken to control the disorder cause gingival hypoplasia. Make any restorations fixed and strong so that they are not dislodged during a seizure. Consult the child's medical practitioner to discover the frequency of seizures, their precipitating factors and the drug regimen.

Epileptic fit: see Chapter 11.

Chapter 13

Some oral and dental diseases of childhood

Predeciduous teeth have been reported on rare occasions. They are small, weakly attached to the mucosa and need to be differentiated from prematurely erupting primary teeth. They are usually extracted to avoid breast feeding difficulties.

Bohn's nodules (Epstein's pearls; dental lamina cyst of the newborn). Small, white, raised nodules found sometimes on the alveolar ridge or at the junction of the hard and soft palates. They are formed from epithelial remnants of the dental lamina or retained in the line of fusion of the palate. They do not cause any symptoms and resolve spontaneously or at the time of tooth eruption. No treatment is necessary.

Teething

Signs and symptoms

Systemic
The child is irritable, cries a lot, keeps putting its fingers into its mouth and suffers disturbed sleep (which also upsets the rest of the family). The appetite will be reduced but there is increased thirst.

Local
The child may have a red cheek on the affected side and spots around the mouth together with excessive salivation and dribbling. In the mouth there is acute local inflammation over the erupting tooth and the gum is red, swollen and tender.

Treatment

Local
Give the child smooth, clean, hard objects to bite on. Water-filled 'Teethers' (from Mothercare shops, etc.), cooled in a refrigerator before use, can be very effective. Rusks will also help.

Topical
Oral sugar-free choline salicylate dental gel e.g. Bonjela or Teejel, can be applied every 3–4 hours before food and at bedtime, to relieve pain.

(Note: Excessive use of these gels may cause salicylate poisoning. However, the recent warnings on the link between aspirin and Reye's disease does not apply to non-aspirin salicylates or topical application of teething gels.)

General
Analgesics may be given, e.g Paracetamol elixir paediatric or Calpol infant suspension.

Sedatives such as chloral or dichloralphenazone elixirs have been recommended by some authorities to restore the baby's sleeping cycle and to give the parents some rest. *But* if the pain is relieved, the child will sleep well and it is dangerous to sedate tiny children at any time.

Reassure the parents that the condition is normal and will resolve in time.

Eruption cysts

Signs and symptoms

These are an occasional complication of teething, usually seen over erupting molars. The space over the crown fills with tissue fluid and blood and shows as a dark-bluish tense area sometimes surrounded by inflammation.

Treatment

Eruption cysts usually resolve themselves. This may be assisted with the usual teething aids: rusks, 'Teethers'.

In rare cases it may be necessary to open the cyst under local anaesthesia, cutting away an oval of tissue from the roof of the cyst to expose the crown of the underlying tooth.

Developmental defects

Developmental defects of the teeth and oral structures may be due to hereditary factors or to infection or metabolic disturbances during pregnancy or infancy.

A. Tooth number

Congenital absence of teeth or supernumerary teeth can occur fairly commonly.

Missing teeth

Anodontia.   A total non-development of the teeth due to aplasia of the dental lamina. The condition may be associated with ectodermal dysplasia when, in addition to the absence of all teeth, the child may have a dry skin with an absence of sweat glands, sparse thin hair and eyebrows, and defects of the fingernails. The dental deficiencies can be overcome by the construction of dentures at an early stage and future dental care remains a prosthetic problem. The dentures have to be remade from time to time to ensure facial growth.

Hypodontia.   A developmental absence of some of the teeth that again may be associated with ectodermal dysplasia. The teeth that are present may be malformed, but should be retained wherever possible to form the basis of partial dentures and bridgework. Great efforts must be made to achieve good oral hygiene and preventive care from an early stage to protect the few teeth that are present.

Occasionally, teeth are found not to have developed in otherwise normal children, commonly the upper lateral incisors, the second premolars or the third molars. Missing third molars present no particular difficulty, but the other teeth can give rise to problems with regard to aesthetics and spacing which may need an orthodontist's help and advice. A decision has to be made about closing the incisor space or maintaining it for possible bridgework later. Non-formation of the premolar may mean that it is necessary to retain the primary second molar into adult life.

It is always advisable to check radiographically that all the unerupted permanent teeth are forming properly before extracting the primary predecessors.

Where a tooth is missing from the arch and there is no history of extraction a radiograph will confirm its absence or unerupted presence. Impeded eruption or impaction may have occurred.

Supernumerary teeth

These are usually found in the incisor (90% of cases), premolar, and occasionally molar regions. Their presence in the primary dentition does not always predict a similar condition in the permanent teeth. They tend to cause orthodontic problems and commonly require early extraction.

B. Tooth structure

Dentinogenesis imperfecta (hereditary opalescent dentine)
Hereditary defect of dentine formation which may be associated with other mesodermal tissue defects, e.g. osteogenesis imperfecta.

Type I Inherited (dominant trait) in families in association with osteogenesis imperfecta.

Type II Inherited (dominant trait) without association with osteogenesis imperfecta.

Deciduous teeth are usually severely affected and in Type II the permanent teeth are as well. The teeth are discoloured opalescent grey-blue to yellow-brown. The enamel is soon fractured away under occlusal stress and the underlying dentine wears down quickly occlusally until the pulp of the teeth may be exposed.

Radiographically the teeth show early obliteration of the pulp chambers and often short roots.

Treatment is aimed at preventing the loss of tooth tissue. Early application of stainless steel crowns on the posterior teeth and cast crowns for the adult teeth are indicated. Adhesive cements such as glass-ionomers can help short-term in some cases. Problems arise in restorative treatment because of the extremely soft structure of the crowns and roots.

Amelogenesis imperfecta
Hereditary defect of enamel formation not associated with other general defects. The condition is confined to tissue with epithelial ectodermal origins and thus the underlying mesodermal dentine is normal.

The defect may be:

Hypoplastic: thin enamel.
Hypocalcified: soft enamel.
Hypomatured: chips away easily from the dentine.

Radiographs show enamel deficiences, thinness and reduced radiodensity in most cases. The shape of the tooth is often normal.

Enamel hypoplasia
Other forms of defective enamel formation may be:

1. Inherited (usually a dominant trait), or
2. Environmental: e.g. due to fevers, local infections, congenital syphilis etc., drugs, excess fluorides.

The effects may be localized to a particular period of the tooth development and this may give a valuable clue in discovering the environmental cause.

Usually the part of the tooth formed *in utero* is protected and sound except in rare inherited cases of hypoplasia. As primary teeth are shed diagnosis can be helped by examining them under the microscope. The junction between prenatal and postnatal enamel is indicated by the neonatal line or ring histologically.

It is not always possible to identify environmental causes of enamel hypoplasia because of inadequate information and when the parent has a poor memory of the medical history.

Tetracycline teeth: The broad-spectrum antibiotic tetracycline is bound to calcium and deposited in growing bones and teeth. Affected teeth are disfigured by bands of discoloration ranging from grey to dark orange-brown. This drug should not be given to children under 12 years of age or to pregnant women.

Fluorosis: Excessively high levels of fluoride ingested during enamel formation can cause enamel fluorosis with varying degrees of white or brown patches of discoloration on the affected teeth.

Dental caries

Definition

Dental caries is a microbial disease of the calcified structures of the teeth which demineralizes the inorganic component and destroys the organic substance of the tooth structure.

Aetiology

At present the causation of dental caries is still best explained by the multifactorial model: susceptible tooth + caries potential microflora + a suitable substrate + time. Plaque bacteria produce acid by fermenting ingested refined carbohydrates, especially sugars. This acid causes demineralization of the enamel surface and if the process is not checked will result in progressive destruction of the tooth. Predisposing factors include a frequent high sugar intake in the diet, poor oral hygiene, reduced access to fluoride, and aspects such as the quality and quantity of salivary flow. Effective control can only be achieved through an approach based on prevention using relatively simple preventive methods.

Pathology

The full pathology of dental caries is not included here, but certain aspects are important in the prevention and early diagnosis of the disease in children.

When white spot lesions are examined under the scanning electron microscope it can be shown that organisms can have penetrated to the full depth of the enamel and even into the dentine even before there is a gross loss of tooth substance. Studies have shown that the decalcification of the carious lesion at this stage is an ebb and flow process and thus remineralization can take place given a change in the disease-promoting environment.

Other studies have shown that where communication between the organisms and the oral cavity has been blocked, i.e. by fissure sealing the surface, then the organisms are deprived of nutrition and gradually killed.

In recent years the changing caries experience, perhaps associated with the almost universal use of fluoride toothpastes, has demanded a special vigilance when searching for lesions. Twenty years ago cariously undermined enamel broke away easily under occlusal stresses and the patient was rapidly aware of a sharp edge, food impaction and pain. The modern caries attack is usually much slower and does not usually result in a rapid structural failure of the tooth. This can lead to the occurrence of 'occult caries' in the 'fluoride tooth' where a stronger enamel structure can conceal deep caries that may extend and 'mushroom' asymptomatically into dentine via a fissure or pit that outwardly appears to be minimally stained.

Diagnosis

On examination teeth must be dried well and viewed with a good light and preferably under magnification. Fissures may be tested gently with a probe, although it must be recognized that heavy pressure with a sharp probe on a white spot lesion can damage the decalcified structure to such an extent that there is no hope of remineralization and repair. Cavities may also be detected by a fibreoptic light terminal placed against one wall of the tooth so that the carious lesion may be detected by the lack of light conduction. Small fibreoptic points for interproximal illumination are available and good results have been reported.

Standard bite-wing radiographs can be taken when necessary to monitor suspected surfaces in posterior teeth. The films should be examined with great care, preferably with a variable light source and under magnification. As well as checking the contact point areas it is important to look specifically at the areas beneath the occlusal fossa in molar teeth.

Diagnostic methods in the future may include testing the tooth by electrical resistance, better imaging methods, and computerized radiograph analysis.

The need for accurate diagnosis and assessment of dental caries becomes imperative in order that the dentist can decide which lesions require operative treatment and which deserve to be kept under observation. A decade ago to leave a stained, 'sticky' fissure unopened and unfilled would have amounted to negligence. Now careful judgement is required in planning treatment for a carious tooth to decide whether to fill a particular lesion, to investigate it or to wait and 'give prevention time to work'.

Rampant caries

This is a condition in which the patient suffers an acute onset of rapidly destructive lesions involving most of the erupted teeth. These can occur on surfaces usually immune to decay and soon progress to involve the dental pulp. In the primary dentition it is usually found in upper incisors and the molar teeth and, commonly though not always, associated with incorrect use of infant feeding bottles, sugared comforters, sugar-based medicines and other dietary problems. In the permanent dentition the teeth are affected as they erupt into the same oral environment and thus they can follow the same problem in the primary dentition.

The aetiology of rampant caries is obscure, but it is thought that diet, inadequate oral hygiene techniques, salivary factors, and the surface texture and morphology of the teeth themselves may play a part.

Periodontal disease

(Any disease peculiar to the periodontium. Usually taken to mean inflammatory lesions of the gingiva and tooth-supporting structures.)

Periodontal disease in children has received little attention until comparatively recently, but interest is now being aroused with the realization that the foundations of chronic conditions in adults may be laid in the young patient. Early recognition of periodontal disease is vitally important so that suitable preventive treatment can be instituted before irreversible damage has occurred.

Marginal gingivitis

Prevalence

This is the commonest periodontal disorder in children in both the primary and permanent dentitions, while periodontitis is uncommon.

Various figures of prevalence up to 87% have been given for children in many published surveys and these show the condition to be more severe in many Asian and African countries than in the USA or Scandinavia. Comparisons are made more difficult because of the different diagnostic criteria and methods of assessment that were used. However, more recently adopted methods of indices and standard criteria and standardization of examiners should provide better methods for the basis of comparison.

It appears that while some children have gingivitis before the age of 6 years, after this age there is a great increase in numbers reaching a temporary peak (puberty gingivitis) at 11 years in girls and 13 years in boys. In young children gingivitis very rarely leads to irreversible periodontal changes. From age 13 onwards the proportion with periodontal pockets and alveolar bone loss increases and the prevalence of periodontal disease appears to follow a linear progression from adolescence to old age. Subjects from groups with higher living standards and educational levels are said to have lower prevalence—perhaps due to better oral hygiene and more awareness of oral health values.

Appearance

Instead of the firm stippled appearance of the healthy gingivae, in marginal gingivitis there is an inflammatory response so that they are red at the marginal zone with loss of stippling, and the papillae may bleed at the slightest touch. The condition may be localized to a single papilla or it may extend to include many. The most commonly affected regions are the anterior segments.

Aetiology

Gingivitis may be due to local oral causes, systemic factors or oral habits.

Local causes include:

1. Plaque. This is the soft, non-mineralized bacterial deposit which forms on inadequately cleaned teeth. There appears to be a direct association between gingivitis and the presence of plaque on the necks of the teeth. The toxic products of the bacteria in the plaque produce an irritant response in the

gingivae resulting in chronic inflammation. Although plaque is constantly forming and can never be entirely eliminated the associated gingivitis improves when the oral hygiene standards improve and sufficient plaque is removed daily to keep its level below the pathological threshold which causes the inflammatory response. Gross caries, poor restorations, orthodontic appliances and dentures all contribute to plaque retention.

2. Calculus is found occasionally in young children. When it is present the calculus is not in direct contact with the gingiva but separated from it by a layer of soft plaque. The presence of calculus is an indication of poor oral hygiene and in itself produces even poorer oral cleansing because it hinders effective tooth brushing.

3. Tooth eruption. The increased prevalence of gingivitis from 6 years of age and later may be associated with tooth eruption. The gingiva adjacent to an erupting tooth shows some enlargement and rounding, but this reverts to a more normal appearance when the tooth comes into occlusion and function, unless other causes of gingivitis are operating.

4. Local disease. Tenderness or pain in a tooth causes a disinclination to use that side of the mouth, and plaque and food debris collect. This is seen frequently around the area of a loose exfoliating deciduous tooth and tends to remain localized and to disappear when the cause is removed.

5. Malocclusion. Irregular and malpositioned teeth tend to predispose towards localized gingivitis.

6. Mouth breathing. A more hypoplastic type of gingivitis occurs in patients who mouth breathe. True mouth breathing can be distinguished from open mouth posture by checking nose and mouth with a wisp of cotton wool to detect air movement. The constant movement of air over the gingivae dries the surface of the tissues and allows the accumulation of irritating debris without it being washed over by saliva. Treatment generally requires consultation with an ENT specialist to check the nasopharynx for enlarged adenoids etc., a careful oral hygiene regime and daily protection of the gingivae by the local application of petroleum jelly to prevent dehydration. In some cases the construction of an oral screen, worn in labial vestibule at night, may be indicated in order to break the habit.

Systemic causes include:

1. Puberty. The hormonal changes at puberty are thought to make the oral tissues more susceptible to gingival irritation and that

gingivitis already present to a lesser degree is exacerbated to a peak at puberty.

2. Diabetes mellitus. Patients with undiagnosed or uncontrolled diabetes have an exaggerated gingival response to local irritants. In a child with chronic gingivitis of which the severity appears to be greater than expected from local causes, diabetes is a possibility to be investigated by urine tests.

3. Haematological disorders. If the chronic gingivitis presents any atypical features further advice from a physician should be sought in case the condition may be the oral manifestation of such diseases as leukaemia, neutropenia, or agranulocytosis, etc.

4. Immunosuppressant drug therapy.

5. Down's syndrome children tend to be predisposed to gingival inflammation and subsequent periodontitis.

Gingival enlargement

This may arise as a result of:

1. Chronic inflammation.

2. Drug therapy. Phenytoin (Epanutin) taken to control epileptic seizures.

3. Hereditary gingival fibromatosis: Rare genetic syndrome in which gingival enlargement is a feature. There is little local inflammation in the firm gingival tissue which tends to completely cover the teeth apart from the occlusal surfaces and incisal tips.

4. Obscure Sturge–Weber syndrome. An association between an extensive port-wine haemangioma of the upper face and scalp and a similar vascularity of the meninges on the same side, plus spastic hemiparesis. Gingival enlargement is not uncommon.

Local gingival recession

This may occur in children due to such things as:

1. Brushing teeth excessively and incorrectly.

2. Habits leading to self-inflicted injury, e.g. scratching the gum with a fingernail.

3. Orthodontic treatment due to tooth movement or pressure from an appliance.

Acute necrotizing ulcerative gingivitis

This is common in some communities but groups vary from zero in some countries to 10% in 2–6 year olds in Africa. The disease is often associated with stress, poor nutrition, debilitating disease or depression of the host resistance. The patient suffers from episodes of painful localized or general gingivitis with necrosis and ulcers of the interdental papilla and a characteristic halitosis. Each episode can last about a week. Treatment is aimed at gently cleaning the areas of the lesions and instituting a gradual increasingly energetic oral hygiene regime as the condition improves. Where the patient is toxic they should also be given antibiotic treatment with metronidazole or penicillin.

Juvenile periodontitis

This disease has a low prevalence (0.1%), generally in adolescent British schoolchildren. It is thought to be associated with familial, genetic factors, perhaps associated with a neutrophil dysfunction, that lead to an increased susceptibility to periodontal breakdown. Epidemiological studies show ethnic (children of Indian, Middle East or Afro-Caribbean origin) and geographical differences in prevalence and that females tend to be the most commonly affected. The onset of the disease is at puberty and there is extensive destruction of the periodontal tissues, mirrored on both sides of the jaws. Clinically, there is gingival bleeding from apparently normal tissues with little plaque or calculus in evidence. The disease is diagnosed upon radiographic examination. Treatment is by local root planing and systemic tetracycline (250 mg four times a day for two weeks), followed by careful maintenance and monitoring.

Severe alveolar bone destruction may also be found in other diseases such as the rare, hereditary Papillon–Lefèvre syndrome (a dermatological disease characterized by hyperkeratosis of the palms of the hands and the soles of the feet) or in histiocytosis X.

Some disorders of the mucosa

Thrush (Candidiasis)

A fungal (*Candida albicans*) infection causing characteristic adherent white plaques on the buccal mucous membranes and the tongue. It may affect the perineum also. It may occur following prolonged antibiotic therapy or its presence may indicate a defect in the host resistance.

Treatment
Nystatin oral suspension or miconazole oral gel.

Primary herpes simplex

This common viral infection is usually asymptomatic. Less than 10% of infected children become clinically ill. The infecting agent is herpes simplex virus: Virus type 1 is transmitted by infected saliva and causes oral, skin and eye infection, and Virus type 2 causes genital herpes. The infection may be asymptomatic or present as gingivostomatitis.

Acute herpetic gingivostomatitis
(Note: Always wear gloves during examination of a suspected case and discard them afterwards.)

This disorder is very common in pre-school children living in poor socioeconomic conditions. Orally the gingival tissues become inflamed. There is a short prodromal period of itching, before the appearance of small tense vesicles with a reddened base which burst to form ulcers. The ulcers are shallow and painful occurring on the buccal, gingival or pharyngeal mucosa, and red borders of the lips. There is an accompanying fever, irritability, sleep disturbance, pain on swallowing, dribbling and enlarged cervical glands. The ulcers heal in about 7–14 days, completely by 21 days.

Differential diagnosis: Teething, drug eruptions, erythema multiforme, or hand, foot and mouth disease.

Complications: Involvement of the tissues of the vulva or eye. Dehydration. Transmission of the infection to other members of the family. Encephalitis.

Treatment: There is no permanent cure and future recurrences are possible: 'cold sores' related to non-specific factors, e.g. exposure to sunlight. Reassure the parent about the self-limiting nature of the attack.

Symptomatic: Ensure an adequate fluid intake and soft, bland, cool food. Ice can be sucked to relieve the pain. Corsodyl mouthwash applied from time to time with a cotton bud can help to reduce plaque formation if toothbrushing is impossible.

Drug therapy (see Chapter 15).

Systemic: The antiviral drug Acyclovir (Zovirax) can be given in tablet or elixir form five times a day for 5 days.

Topical: Regular topical applications are very difficult to achieve in most cases, for young children.

Acyclovir (Zovirax) cream can be applied to the oral lesions five times a day for 5 days.

Bonjela, Teegel or Orobase ointment applied to the ulcers may reduce the pain at mealtimes.

Tetracycline mouth baths may help older children suffering recurrent herpetic stomatitis.

Hand, foot and mouth disease

A highly contagious, epidemic disease of young children caused by the Coxsackie virus A-16. Incubation period 2–6 days. There is a sudden onset with low-grade fever, sore throat, headache, anorexia and pains in the limbs. The child develops vesicular exanthematous lesions distributed over the buccal mucosa, tongue and hard palate, and similar symptoms on the hands, feet and nappy area. The attack lasts 7–14 days and is self-limiting. (The disease is not related to animal foot and mouth disease.) Differential diagnosis from herpes: hand, foot and mouth disease is much milder and the characteristic rash is on the extremities.

Treatment: Symptomatic. Analgesics and mouthwashes. One attack confers permanent immunity.

Chapter 14

Childhood diseases

A basic knowledge of common childhood diseases and certain special cases is of importance to the dental practitioner for they may present as a diagnostic problem, can occasionally risk being trans-mitted to visitors and members of the staff, and will also have to be taken into account in planning and carrying out treatment for affected children.

Infectious fevers

Prevention

Most of the infectious fevers of childhood are preventable by vaccine immunization.

Immunization schedule

Age	Vaccine	Note
3 months +	Diphtheria Pertussis Tetanus Polio	2nd dose after 6–8 week interval, 3rd dose after 4–6 month interval
12–24 months	Measles	Joined by mumps and rubella from October, 1988
About 5 years	Booster for diphtheria, tetanus and polio	Starting school
10–14 years	Rubella	Girls only
13 years	Tuberculosis	For tuberculin-negative children only
15–19 years	Tetanus Polio	Leaving school, starting work

This complex schedule of immunization is offered to all children in the UK and usually implemented. However, although some 90% of children are immunized, some can still miss the opportunity of being protected for various reasons, e.g. children from abroad, children who were unwell at the time for vaccination, etc., and can present diagnostic and treatment problems in the dental surgery.

Measles (Rubeola)

An acute, infectious viral disease with early catarrh and fever followed by a typical rash. Most contagious by droplet spread in the catarrhal stage. Epidemic in winter and spring; second attacks are rare.

Incubation period
7–14 days.

Symptoms
Photophobia, sneezing, runny nose, conjunctivitis, cough, fever, malaise, Koplik's spots (pin-head size, white, raised on a red base, seen in the buccal mucosa opposite the premolar region). A maculo-papular, irregularly confluent rash appears on the 4th day, starts around the ears and on the face and neck, spreads down the body for 1–2 days and then fades and the patient feels better.

Complications
These include bronchopneumonia or otitis media.

Treatment
Symptomatic. Isolate for 14 days after the rash starts.

Prevention
Vaccines.

German measles (Rubella)

An acute infectious viral disease with fever, glandular enlargement and a typical rash. Probably spread by droplets and close contact. Commonly in the spring. Second attacks are rare.

Incubation period
10–21 days.

Symptoms
Mild cases may pass unnoticed. Onset with headache, sore throat, stiff neck, fever, malaise. There is enlargement of suboccipital, postcervical and mastoid glands. A rash with small, pink macules and papules appears on the 2nd day behind the ears, and on the face, neck, trunk and limbs and fades in 36 hours. Laboratory serological tests may be needed to confirm diagnosis where necessary.

Complications
These are rare in children.

Treatment
Symptomatic.

Prevention
Rubella immunization should be offered to all girls of 13 and women of child-bearing age found to be seronegative.

Special alert
Keep these infected or suspected children away from expectant mothers visiting the surgery. The infection may result in abortion, stillbirth or severe congenital defects (e.g. cardiac, eye, ear, encephalopathy) in children born of mothers infected during early months of pregnancy.

Roseola infantum (Pseudorubella)
An acute disease of young infants probably due to a neurodermotropic virus. Epidemic with an incubation period up to three weeks. Child develops enlarged glands and suffers a high fever which falls immediately as the rubella-like rash appears on about the 4th day. Treatment is symptomatic.

Erythema infectiosum (Fifth Disease)
An acute viral disease of children and adolescents occurring in local outbreaks during the spring with an incubation period of about 10 days. Child develops a low-grade fever, malaise and a confluent erythema on both cheeks which give this disease the name 'slapped cheek syndrome'. The rash spreads to the limbs and body fading to a lacy appearance. The illness lasts about 10 days but can recur over the next few weeks. Treatment is symptomatic.

Scarlet fever (Scarlatina)

This once epidemic and serious illness is less common today probably because the early provision of antibiotic therapy prevents its progress in the individual patient. It is due to infection by certain strains of Group A haemolytic streptococcus which produce an erythrogenic toxin.

Incubation period
3–5 days.

Symptoms
Initially the child complains of a sore throat, with headache, nausea, malaise and fever and on the 2nd day develops a red cutaneous rash affecting most of the body but leaving a characteristic circumoral pallor which stands out against the flushed pink-red face. The rash lasts about 10 days (less with antibiotic therapy) and then in most cases there is a desquamation of the outer layer of the reddened skin especially of the hands and feet. Intra-orally there is first a coated 'white strawberry' tongue followed at desquamation by a 'red strawberry' tongue.

Complications
Rare, but if untreated, otitis media, rheumatic fever, nephritis, etc.

Treatment
Antibiotics for up to 10 days to combat the streptococcal infection.

Chicken pox (Varicella)

An acutely infectious viral disease, spread by droplets, fomites (infected clothing, bedding, etc.) and through the air, with fever and a typical vesicular rash. Cases occur in winter and spring.

Incubation period
11–21 days.

Symptoms
Onset: headache, malaise, shivering, fever. Rash appears in crops after 2–7 days and runs a course through macules, papules, vesicles and pustules. It is denser in the centre of the body appearing on the trunk, face, scalp, and limbs, and also on the mucosa of the cheeks, palate and pharynx. The lesions burst and crust over to form scabs within a few days and these then take over a week to separate, leaving a white scar.

Complications
Secondary infection of the vesicles.

Treatment
Symptomatic. Rest. Avoid scratching. Soothing lotions. Prevent and treat secondary infection of the vesicles with antibiotics.

Prevention
Isolate the patient until the last scab has separated. Usually after about 14 days after the rash started. Vaccines.

Whooping cough (Pertussis)

An acute communicable bacterial disease (*B. pertussis*) with paroxysmal bouts of coughing usually ending by a prolonged crowing inspiration or whoop. Most common in the spring.

Incubation period
6–18 days.

Symptoms
Begins with a cold and cough. In about 10 days it reaches the paroxysmal stage with a noisy, explosive, rapidly repeated, expiratory cough, even to the point of cyanosis and tears, followed by the characteristic inspiratory whoop and occasionally leading to vomiting. The cough follows any exertion and is worse at night. Diagnosis is confirmed by culture of the *B. pertussis* from a nasopharyngeal swab. The child will have congested conjunctivae, a slightly swollen face and may have an ulcer under the tongue from friction with the teeth while coughing. This spasmodic stage lasts about 2 weeks and then becomes less severe although the child may have a cough for many weeks.

Complications
Include bronchopneumonia and hernia.

Treatment
Symptomatic. Rest.

Prevention
Isolate patient for at least 4 weeks. Vaccine given in the 'triple vaccine' along with diphtheria and tetanus vaccines.

Mumps (Epidemic parotitis)

An acute infectious generalized viral disease with painful enlargement of the salivary glands due to hyperaemia of the connective tissue. Generally the parotid glands are affected. Epidemic in winter and spring.

Incubation period
14–18 days.

Symptoms
Headache, malaise, sore throat, fever, swelling of one of the parotid glands with fullness behind the angle of the mandible spreading in front of the ear and down into the neck. It is difficult to feel the jaw through the swelling. Commonly the other side is soon affected. The mouth is dry, there is an increased pain on chewing and swallowing, especially with acidic foods that stimulate salivation. The symptoms usually resolve in about a week.

Complications
Include orchitis (sterility is rare) and pancreatitis.

Treatment
Bed rest, soft diet and analgesics.

Prevention
Isolate the patient for 14 days, watch susceptible contacts. Vaccine.

Diphtheria

An acute contagious disease caused by *Corynebacterium diphtheriae*. Present in the nose and throat of affected patients and carriers.

Incubation period
2–6 days.

Symptoms
Tiredness, mild sore throat gradually proceeding to more serious malaise and fever. A white to grey-green membrane appears on the tonsils and the neck glands soon swell extensively even to produce the 'bull neck' of severe diphtheria.

Complications
Oedema of the larynx or infection extending into the trachea can

cause respiratory complications. Cardiovascular collapse and various nerve paralyses (e.g. eye, pharynx, larynx, respiration) due to toxins can occur.

Treatment
Antitoxin and antibiotics. Hospitalize and isolate. Observe and immunize contacts.

Prevention
Diphtheria is a preventable disease. Vaccine given in 'triple vaccine' regime along with tetanus and whooping cough vaccines.

Glandular fever (Infectious mononucleosis)

An acute disease of adolescence caused by the Epstein–Barr virus with high fever, sore throat and generalized glandular enlargement. Not very contagious.

Incubation period
4–6 weeks.

Symptoms
Include malaise, fatigue, headache, shivering, fever, cough, sore throat, and generalized glandular enlargement. The liver and spleen may be affected. The eyelids may swell. There may be a transient rash which may be precipitated by ampicillin therapy. Blood and serological tests are needed to confirm the diagnosis. Differential diagnosis can be difficult. Recovery is usual within 1–2 weeks, although weakness and fatigue may be prolonged.

Treatment
There is no specific treatment. Symptomatic, with bed rest during the acute phase of malaise and fever.

Tetanus (Lockjaw)

An acute disease due to wound infection with the spore-forming tetanus bacillus (*Clostridium tetani*) which is commonly present in soil and the intestines of animals such as the horse and the cow.

Incubation period
Usually 2–12 days but may be as long as 50 days.

Symptoms
Violent, painful and exhausting muscular spasms. Usually the disease first attacks the muscles of the face and jaw and then spreads to the rest of the body, causing dysphagia, laryngeal and respiratory spasm and arching of the back. The prognosis is poor if initiation and progress of the disease is rapid.

Treatment
Hospitalize. Sedation. Respiratory support. Human antitetanus immune globulin (HTIG).

Prevention
Tetanus is a preventable disease. Active immunization gives complete protection. The vaccine is given in the 'triple vaccine' (see Immunization Schedules) and gives protection in childhood and basic immunity for booster doses of tetanus vaccine at school age or after a potentially tetanus-contaminated wound. Such an injury requires careful cleaning and antibiotic therapy. Early administration of vaccine elicits a protective antibody level in a previously immunized patient. If the wounded patient is inadequately immunized then they should be given human antitetanus globulin plus a first injection of vaccine. Arrangements must be made for the 2nd and 3rd doses of vaccine to be given at monthly intervals subsequently.

Skin diseases

Acne

A common inflammatory disease of the skin with inflamed nodules, papules, pustules, etc. on the face, neck and upper thorax. It is due to physiological adjustment of sebaceous glands to hormone changes of puberty and in adolescence. It may have psychological effects on the teenager who is sensitive about his appearance.

Treatment
Locally to remove the pore plugs. Systemically: administration of long-term low dose antibiotics (e.g. tetracycline 250 mg twice a day).

Head lice

An infestation common in schoolchildren. The lice live on the scalp and lay tiny white eggs (nits) which stick to the hair. Can be transmitted by close contact of heads, etc. The bites of the lice do not appear to transmit disease, but cause a persistent itch and secondary dermatitis.

Treatment
Malathon solution, 0.5%, special shampoos and fine-tooth combing of the hair.

Impetigo

A highly contagious superficial skin infection which progresses rapidly through the small pimple or vesicular phase to form typical golden-brown crusty scabs. Impetigo spreads very rapidly and needs early effective treatment. The causative organism is usually a haemolytic streptococcus although *Staphylococcus aureus* is frequently cultured from these lesions.

Treatment
Chlortetracycline hydrochloride cream, 3%, applied locally and a systemic antibiotic.

Ringworm

A very contagious fungus infection which affects the skin and sometimes the fingernails. Scaly, crusted lumps form with a clear centre and spread out from the site of infection. In the scalp, the hair breaks off in the affected area.

Treatment
Topical antifungal preparation.

Scabies

A mite spread by close family contact. Invades the horny layer of the skin and lays eggs. Burrows in the hands, wrists, elbows, feet and face. Lesions itch badly.

Treatment
Benzyl benzoate emulsion painted on the skin, etc.

Warts (Verrucae)

Common, contagious, rough excrescences on the skin caused by a papovirus. Many children get them. They are harmless and self-limiting and generally disappear spontaneously.

Treatment
Treated only if they are painful and then by curetting or freezing with liquid nitrogen, etc.

Chapter 15

Prescribing for children

Calculating dosages

Several methods have been suggested for calculating the doses of a drug appropriate for a child, and these are based upon the child's age, body weight or body surface area.

Age

Calculations based upon the child's age to determine the fraction of the adult dose can give differing results.

Young's Rule: Child's age/age + 12.

Cushing's Rule: Child's age/24.

Body weight

Clark's Rule divides the child's body weight in pounds by 150 to arrive at the fraction of the adult dose, e.g. for a child of 50 lb 50/150 = ⅓ of the adult dose. This method may lead to an overdose in a very obese child.

Body surface area

The most reliable method uses an assessment of the child's body surface area in square metres, expressed as a fraction of that of 1.8 sq m for a 70-kg adult, to arrive at the appropriate proportion of the adult dose. The body surface area can be calculated, given the child's height and weight, from paediatric tables (nomograms). Approximate values can be found in the current edition of the *British National Formulary* and the more accurate nomogram in several publications, for example, in Insley, J. (1986) *A Paediatric Vade-Mecum*, 11th edn, Lloyd-Luke, London.

From the *British National Formulary:*

Age	Percentage of the adult dose
1	' 25
7	50
12	75

Routes

In dentistry drugs are usually administered topically, orally, by injection, or by inhalation.

Oral preparations are generally preferable to injections of drugs for children. Attention should be given to the timing of oral drug administration for rates of absorption can be affected by ingestion of food. For example, oral penicillin is best taken on an empty stomach about half an hour before food. Conversely, other drugs that may irritate the stomach lining should be taken after food.

Prescribing

When prescribing an unusual item it is wise to always take the time to review its action, side-effects and dosage in a standard reference such as the *British National Formulary* or the *Monthly Index of Medical Specialties (MIMS)*. Sugar-free preparations should be chosen for preference. Particular care must be taken when prescribing for a child with kidney or liver function impairment which will affect the rate at which the drug is excreted from the body, cause toxic reactions, etc. Drugs must remain in the charge of a responsible adult, who should keep them in a secure place out of the child's reach, and generally supervise their administration to avoid non-compliance with instructions or any possibility of the child taking an overdose. Although most drugs are dispensed in child-proof containers many children delight in proving that they can 'solve the puzzle' and open them.

Drug interactions and side-effects

It is important that the prescriber is aware of all the drugs that a child is taking, including those prescribed by other practitioners and self-administered by the parent or child. Drugs should be given for as short a period as possible and drug combinations avoided. The patient's progress must be monitored while they are taking the prescribed drug with regard to the known side-effects and potential drug reactions.

In pregnancy some drugs can cross the placental barrier and affect fetal tissues, e.g. tetracycline and tranquillizers. Drugs can also be passed from mother to child to some extent via breast milk, e.g. salicylates, antibiotics (tetracycline), etc.

Common drugs used in children's dentistry

Analgesics

A child may suffer pain and discomfort of dental origin such as acute pulpitis, dental abscess or traumatic injury, or as a result of oral surgery, etc. Treatment will primarily be directed towards eliminating the cause of pain (e.g. by opening an abscess and administering an antibiotic), but in addition the child may benefit from taking a mild analgesic for a brief period.

Aspirin

Uses: An analgesic and antipyretic.

Contraindications: *Not* suitable for children under the age of 12 years (unless for specific arthritic conditions) because of the link between this drug usage and Reye's syndrome (a severe liver disease with encephalopathy).

Paracetamol

Uses: An analgesic without aspirin's gastrointestinal irritant tendency.

Caution: Avoid prolonged usage or too large a dose because of possible liver damage.

Preparations

Paracetamol Tablets BP	500 mg
Paracetamol Elixir, Paediatric BP	120 mg/5 ml

Calpol (Calmic), Panadol (Winthrop), etc.

Dosage

Up to 1 year	60–120 mg
1–5 years	120–250 mg
6–12 years	250–500 mg

every 6 hours, maximum 4 doses a day only.

Antibiotics

Severe dental infections such as acute dental abscesses causing facial swelling and cellulitis will need systemic antibiotic therapy as well as direct surgical intervention. Prophylactic antibiotic cover will also be required before dental treatment for children with cardiac defects that predispose them to bacterial endocarditis (see Chapter 12).

Before prescribing antibiotics consider:

1. The patient. Have they: (a) any history of sensitivity or allergy to any particular antibiotic, and (b) any physical contraindication to such therapy, e.g. kidney or liver function problems?
2. The infecting organism. E.g. its sensitivity or resistance to a particular antibiotic. For instance viruses will not respond to antibiotics.
3. The route of administration of the antibiotic. In dentistry this will generally be either oral or intramuscular injection.

Penicillin
Used in the treatment of soft-tissue infections and in prophylaxis against bacterial endocarditis.

Benzyl Penicillin (Penicillin G)   is destroyed by gastric juices and in dentistry is given by intramuscular injection. May be used initially to raise the level of antibiotic quickly and is then followed by a suitable oral preparation of penicillin.

Procaine Penicillin   is a slowly soluble salt of Benzyl Penicillin and may be used as an intramuscular depot injection giving satisfactory levels of penicillin for up to 24 hours. Benethamine Penicillin is similar but is only used in combination with other penicillins. Penicillin Triple inj. BPC (Triplopen Glaxo) contains benethamine penicillin, procaine penicillin and benzylpenicillin all in powder form ready to be reconstituted with 'water for injection'.

Phenoxymethyl Penicillin (Penicillin V)   is stable through the stomach and used for oral administration. It is available in tablets, capsules or syrups (the latter have a limited life of 7 days once they have been made up). It should be taken at least half an hour before food.

Caution: Check for history of sensitivity or kidney impairment.

Side-effects: May give rise to sensitivity reactions (skin rash, joint pains, oedema, respiratory effects, anaphylactic shock). Oral penicillin may cause diarrhoea.

Dosage: Must be based on the severity of the particular infection and continued long enough to gain a response from that infection and to avoid resistant strains developing. Adult doses usually range from 250 mg to 500 mg. The drug is given every 6 hours generally and in most dental cases a course of 4 to 8 days is enough.

Broad-spectrum penicillin

Amoxycillin: Derived from Ampicillin, and better absorbed when taken orally, is unaffected by the presence of food in the stomach.

Uses: Oral treatment of soft-tissue infections.

Caution: Check for a history of sensitivity to penicillin. Note that in cases of glandular fever and leukaemia a maculopapular rash may develop that is not considered to be due to penicillin allergy.

Contraindication: Sensitivity to penicillin.

Preparations: Amoxycillin capsules BP 250 mg. Proprietary Amoxil Capsules. Amoxycillin Mixture BP 250 mg/5 ml. Proprietary Amoxil Syrup (sugar free). Amoxycillin oral powder. Amoxil sachets 750 mg and 3 g.

Dose: Adult 250 mg/8 hours.
Under 10 years 125 mg/8 hours (*see* Chapter 12).

Tetracyclines
These are broad-spectrum antibiotics which should not be given systemically to children under 12 years of age or to expectant mothers because they are deposited in developing and growing teeth and bones and will cause irreversible staining and hypoplasia of enamel (see tetracyline mouth baths in the Treatment of Mouth Ulcers later).

Erythromycin: Similar antibiotic effects to penicillin and may be used in cases of penicillin sensitivity.

Contraindication: In cases of liver impairment.

Side-effects: Nausea, vomiting, and diarrhoea with large doses.

Preparation: Erythromycin stearate tablets BP 250 mg/tablet.
Erythromycin succinate suspensions (Proprietary Erythroped
(Abbott)) are offered in a choice of strengths ranging from 125 mg/
5 ml to 500 mg/5 ml. Life of diluted syrup is 5 days.

Dose: Orally 250–500 mg/6 hours.
Child 125–250 mg/6 hours. (*see* Chapter 12).

Antifungal drugs

Nystatin
Used in the treatment of oral and perioral *Candida albicans*
infections (Thrush; Candidiasis).

Preparations: Nystatin mixture BP intraoral.
100 000 units/ml. Put 1 ml in the mouth and retain it near the lesion
4 times a day, after meals, and continue for 3 days after the lesions
have healed.

Nystatin ointment. For perioral lesions.
100 000 units/g. Apply 2–4 times a day and continue for a week
after the lesions have healed.

Treatment of mouth ulcers

Acyclovir (Zovirax)
Used in the treatment of herpes simplex infections of skin and
mucous membranes.

Contraindications: Kidney impairment cases should be given a
reduced dose. Some patients may become hypersensitive to acyclovir.

Side-effects: May sometimes cause mild side-effects. Skin rashes
and gastrointestinal tract effects have been reported.

Preparations: 200 mg tabs. 200 mg/5 ml suspension. Banana
flavoured. 5% cream in an aqueous base for skin lesions.

Dosage: 200 mg acyclovir given 5 times a day at 4-hourly intervals
omitting the night-time dose. Treatment continued for 5 days. In
severe cases the course of treatment may have to be extended.

Children over 2 years should have the full adult dose. Below 2 years half adult dose in suspension.

Carmellose sodium (Orabase (Squibb))
A gel which provides mechanical protection when applied over oral lesions before meals.

Corticosteroids
Applied to oral lesions will reduce inflammation. Not to be used in the presence of untreated oral infection. Triamcinolone acetonide (Adcortyl (Squibb)) in Orabase: to be applied thinly to the lesions 2–4 times a day.

Hydrocortisone 2.5 mg pellets (Corlan (Glaxo)): One pellet to be dissolved slowly in the mouth adjacent to the lesion 4 times a day.

Tetracycline mouth baths
Used to treat severe primary and recurrent herpetic ulceration. 10 ml of tetracyline hydrochloride mixture containing 250 mg tetracyline are held in the mouth for 2–3 min, 3 times a day for 3 days. The mixture must not be swallowed. This treatment requires a 3-day break after 3 days of mouth baths to avoid the occurrence of oral thrush.

Salicylates
Choline Salicylate Dental Gel (Bonjela (R & C), Teegel (Napp)) are flavoured gels which are to be rubbed gently on to the lesions before meals and at bedtime. (Note: The warning about the association between aspirin and Reye's syndrome does not apply to non-aspirin salicylate dental gels.)

Chlorhexidine gluconate
1% in a gel brushed on the teeth twice a day, or 0.2% in a mouthwash used 4 times a day will improve oral hygiene, reduce plaque scores and promote healing in cases of oral infection particularly where toothbrushing is impossible. Some reversible staining of the teeth may occur.

Anxiolytics, sedatives and hypnotics

Chloral hydrate
A hypnotic drug used for insomnia which can calm a young child for dental treatment. It has an unpleasant taste which needs to be masked in children's elixirs and for adults an encapsulated form is preferred.

Side-effect: May cause gastrointestinal disturbance.

Preparation: Chloral elixir, paediatric 200 mg/5 ml.

Dose: Insomnia: 30–50 mg per kg of weight up to a maximum single dose of 1 g, well diluted with water to reduce gastric irritation. Sedation: 250 mg 3 times daily.

Dichloralphenazone
Similar to chloral hydrate but with fewer gastrointestinal disturbances.

Preparation: Welldorm (S & N Pharm) Elixir 225 mg/5 ml.

Dose: 1–5 years 225–450 mg; 6–12 years 450–900 mg, well diluted in water.

Benzodiazepines
These have a low incidence of adverse effects and may be classified as:

Short Acting (from 6 to 24 hours) when administered in moderate doses, with few residual effects next day, e.g. Temazepam.

Intermediate to Long Acting (more than 24 hours). With these drugs the effect persists and repeated doses can accumulate in the tissues, e.g. Diazepam.

Temazepam
A short-acting, rapid onset drug useful for teenagers rather than young children.

Dose: Adult, 10–30 mg taken orally an hour before operation produce sedative effects that will last 1–2 hours.

Preparations: Temazepam capsules 10 mg; Temazepam elixir 10 mg/5 ml (life of elixir 14 days).

Diazepam
Is an anxiolytic, sedative and hypnotic. Its use affects the patient's ability to drive (or ride a bicycle) or operate machinery and in certain cases may make them feel drowsy, confused, giddy or faint. The effect may persist for over 24 hours after a single dose.

Preparations: For oral administration the drug is produced in capsule, tablet, syrup and elixir forms of various strengths. Diazepam; Valium (Roche).

Dose: For anxiety, Adult dose up to 30 mg daily: Children 1–5 mg/day in divided doses. For oral sedation in children: up to 15 mg/day taken in divided doses.

Although this drug has been commonly recommended in the literature for some time, its effect is not always predictable when prescribed short term, perhaps in a single dose, for mild anxiety in children. This may be partially explained by the reasons mentioned in the introduction to this section, such as the factors affecting the rate of absorption. However, one recent study found oral diazepam to be ineffective for sedating children up to the age of 13 in the dental surgery. Nevertheless, the drug is generally found to be effective for teenage children and adults in whom paradoxical reactions are less common.

Diazepam may also be administered with satisfactory effects by i.m. and i.v. injection for sedation. This is not recommended for children as a routine procedure but is used occasionally in specialist centres with trained staff and adequate recovery facilities.

Antihistamines

Antihistamines are used in the treatment of allergies, etc. and many also have a sedative and hypnotic effect. Among those suggested for sedating anxious children are Promethazine (Phenergan (M & B)) and Trimeprazine tartrate (Vallergan (M & B)).

Norms

Temperature

A child's temperature may be taken in the mouth, the armpit (axilla) or the rectum. In the dental surgery the temperature is usually taken in the mouth but for small children the axilla might be chosen. Do not attempt to take the temperature if the child has just eaten or drunk anything, has an inflamed mouth or has engaged in violent activity like running. Rinse the thermometer in cold water and wipe it dry. Check that a glass thermometer has been shaken down or that an electric thermometer is switched on and functioning properly.

The mouth
Place the thermometer tip under the child's tongue, and then keep the mouth closed.

The axilla
Make sure the skin is dry and that the bulb of the thermometer is in close contact with two skin surfaces and that all air is excluded.

Leave the thermometer in position for an appropriate time (usually one minute but check because thermometers vary).

Remove the thermometer, note the temperature, then shake down, or switch off the thermometer, wash it in cold soapy water or alcohol and store it dry.

Normal body temperature is about 37°C, but it can vary even in healthy children and may normally be 36.5°C or 37.5°C, and will change during the day, and as a result of activity, excitement or emotion such as crying. A temperature over 37.8°C indicates fever and 40°C indicates a high fever.

Pulse and respiration

The arterial pulse, which reflects the heart beat, may be felt at the radial artery in the wrist or the temporal artery just in front of the ear. As a rule the ratio of the pulse to respiration rate is 4 to 1. The resting pulse rate rises with exercise or excitement or with emotion such as anger, anxiety or fear. In fever the rate increases by approximately five beats per °C as the temperature rises above normal.

Normal respiration is regular, quiet and rhythmical. Its rate like the pulse, rises during exercise, excitement, emotion and fever.

Normal pulse and respiration rates per minute

	Pulse	*Respiration*
Newborn	80–160	20–40
1 year	110–140	about 30
2–5 years	about 100	22–28
6–10 years	about 95	19–22
11–13 years	about 90	about 19
14 years	about 70	about 18
Adult	65–80	16–18

Tooth development dates

(Based on the work of Aitchison (1940))

Primary dentition (Figures A.1–A.5)

	Starts *(in utero)*	*Calcification* *Completed*	*Erupts*	*Resorption* *Starts*	*Tooth* *Shed*
A B	18 weeks	18 months	6 months 8 months	3 years before the tooth is shed	7 years 8 years
D	20 weeks	20 months	12 months		9 years
C E	24 weeks	24 months	18 months 24 months		11 years 10 years

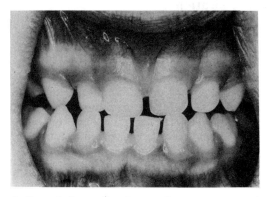

Figure A.1 Sound primary incisor teeth and supporting structures at age 4 years

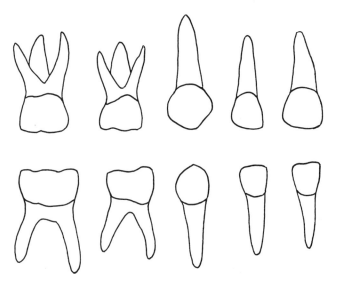

Figure A.2 Anatomy of the primary teeth

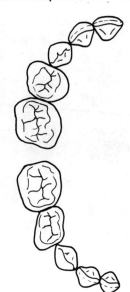

Figure A.3 Occlusal anatomy of the primary teeth

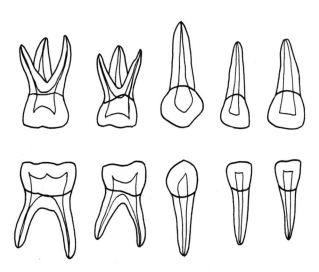

Figure A.4 Pulp anatomy of the primary teeth

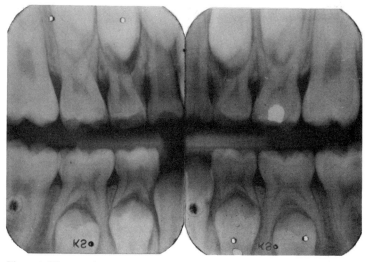

Figure A.5 Intraoral radiograph of primary molars

Permanent dentition

		Upper	Lower	Calcification	
1	1st incisor	7	6.5	Begins 6 years	Completed
2	2nd incisor	8	7.5	before eruption	3 years after
3	canine	11	11	*except* the	eruption *except*
4	1st premolar	9	10	canine and 3rd	the canine and
5	2nd premolar	10	11	molar which	3rd molar which
6	1st molar	6	6	begin 9 years	are fully calcified
7	2nd molar	12	12	before eruption	on eruption
8	3rd molar	17–24	17–24		

Each permanent tooth takes approximately 9 years to calcify and erupts into the mouth about 3 years before completion (except the canines and 3rd molars which are almost fully calcified upon eruption). A tooth takes about 9 years to calcify from crown to apex. The crown takes 3 years, and the root takes 6 years. From this one can estimate fairly accurately the stage of development of an individual tooth at a particular age. The teeth of the female erupt slightly earlier than the male. The first permanent molar starts to calcify about one month before birth.

For example:
The permanent upper central incisor:

Erupts at 7 years, ⅔ completed
Calcification completed   7 years + 3 = 10 years
Calcification commenced 10 years − 9 = 1 year
Crown fully calcified   1 year + 3 = 4 years

The permanent upper canine

Erupts at 11 years, fully completed
Calcification commenced 11 years − 9 = 2 years
Crown completed   2 years + 3 = 5 years

Blood tests

Haematological investigations are usually carried out on 4 ml of blood. The commonest information requested by the dental surgeon is for a differential red and white cell count or the bleeding and clotting times. Routine investigations are usually carried out on automated equipment that will provide a printout listing a considerable amount of additional information that needs to be scrutinized.

Normal values

White blood cell count: 4000–11 000/mm^3

Differential white cell count (sometimes expressed in percentages):

Polymorphs   1500–7500/mm^3
Lymphocytes   1000–4500/mm^3
Monocytes   800/mm^3
Eosinophils   400/mm^3
Basophils   200/mm^3

The polymorph count rises in acute infections and falls in the condition of neutropenia. Abnormal primitive cells are seen in leukaemia.

Red blood cell count: 5 000 000/mm^3

Haemoglobin: 14.5 g/100 ml is regarded as 100%, levels vary with age and between mature men and women.

Age	Hb (g/100 ml) (approx.)
0–3 months	19
3–24 months	12
2–13 years	13
Adult male	16 plus/minus 2
Adult female	14 plus/minus 2

Haemoglobin levels fall in anaemias, and such things as chronic illness and bleeding, and rise in polycythaemia and fluid loss e.g. vomiting.

PCV (packed corpuscular volume or haematocrit):   35–54% in men, 30–47% in women and up to 60% in infants.
    It is a test for anaemia or fluid loss.

MCV (mean corpuscular volume), MCH (mean cell haemoglobin), MCHC (mean cell haemoglobin concentration), and MCD (mean cell diameter) are interpreted by specialists in the diagnosis of specific anaemias.

Platelet count: 150 000–350 000/mm^3

A very low platelet count (less than 50 000/mm^3) predisposes inadequate blood clotting and haemorrhage. The platelets are reduced in number in thrombocytopenic purpura, certain anaemias and acute leukaemia, etc., although the platelet count is normal in haemophilia.

Bleeding time: 3–5 minutes

It is increased in leukaemia, purpura and pernicious anaemia. It is normal in haemophilia.

Clotting time: 4–7 minutes

It is increased in haemophilia, Christmas disease, jaundice and if the patient is taking anticoagulant drugs.

Sources and useful addresses

Dental health education sources

British Dental Health Foundation, 88 Gurnards Avenue, Fishermead, Milton Keynes, Buckinghamshire MK6 2AB

British Fluoridation Society Ltd, 63 Wimpole Street, London W1M 8AL

Colgate Professional Services Division, Guildford, Surrey GU2 5LZ (0483 302222)

Crest Professional Services, Proctor and Gamble Ltd, PO Box 1EP, Newcastle upon Tyne NE99 1EP

Dentomax Motivators, Carr House, Carrbottom Road, Bradford BD5 9BJ

General Dental Council Charitable Trust, 37 Wimpole Street, London W1M 8OQ (071 486 2171)

Gibbs Oral Hygiene Service, Hesketh House, Portman Square, London W1A 1DY (071 486 1200)

Health Education Authority, Hamilton House, Mabledon Place, London WC1H 9TZ (071 383 3833)

Johnson and Johnson Dental Care Division, Foundation Park, Roxborough Way, Maidenhead, Berkshire SL6 3UG (062 882 2222)

Minerva Motivators, Minerva Dental Ltd, Courtney House, Oxford Street, Cardiff CF2 3DT

Oral-B, Cooper Health Products, Gatehouse Road, Aylesbury, Bucks HP19 3ED (0296 432601)

Stafford-Miller Ltd, Dental Division, Hatfield, Herts AL10 0NZ

Wisdom, Mouthcare Division, Addis Ltd, Ware Road, Hertford.

Items available range through advice, pamphlets, posters, models, badges, games, samples books, films, computer games, video cassettes and so on. In some cases a charge is made for these materials and there is generally a hire charge for films and videos, which should be reserved well in advance of the date they are needed. New items are constantly being added to the lists.

It is advisable to read and examine carefully all unsolicited 'dental education' material that arrives in the surgery from sources other than those listed above before recommending it to parents and children.

Useful addresses

Asthma Research Council and Asthma Society, 300 Upper Street, London N1 2XX (071 226 2260)

Autistic Society, National, 276 Willesden Lane, London NW2 5RB

Blind, Royal National Institute for the, 224 Great Portland Street, London W1N 6AA (071 388 1266)

Boots 'Healthcare in the Home' catalogue. Any Boots Chemist store in the UK

British Red Cross Society, 9 Grosvenor Crescent, London SW1X 7EJ (071 235 5454)

Childrens' Bureau, National, 8 Wakley Street, Islington, London EC1V 7QE

Cleft Lip and Palate Association, c/o Dental Department, The Hospital for Sick Children, Great Ormond Street, London WC1N 3JH

Deaf, Royal National Institute for the, 105 Gower Street, London WC1E 6AH (071 387 8033)

Department of Health, Portland Court, 158–176 Great Portland Street, London W1N 5DT (071 872 9302)

Disability and Rehabilitation, Royal Association for (RADAR), 25 Mortimer Street, London W1N 8AB (071 637 5400)

Down's Children's Association, National Centre for, 9 Westbourne Road, Edgbaston, Birmingham B15

Epilepsy Association, British, 40 Hanover House, Leeds L23 1BE (0532 439393)

Epilepsy, National Society for, Chalfont Centre for Epilepsy, Chalfont St Peter, Gerrards Cross, Bucks SL9 0RJ (Chalfont St Peter 3991)

Lady Hoare Trust for Physically Disabled Children, 6 North Street, Midhurst, West Sussex GU29 9DJ (073081 3696)

Mentally Handicapped, National Society for (MENCAP), 117–123 Golden Lane, London EC1Y 0RT (071 253 9433)

MIND, National Association for Mental Health, 22 Harley Street, London W1N 2ED (071 637 0741)

National Council for Voluntary Organizations, 26 Bedford Square, London WC1 3HU (071 636 6487)

National Society for the Prevention of Cruelty to Children (NSPCC) Headquarters, 67 Saffron Hill, London EC1N 8RS (071 242 1626)

Sickle Cell Society, Green Lodge, Barretts Green Road, London NW10 (081 961 7795)

Spastics Society, 12 Park Crescent, London W1N 4QE (071 636 5020)

Speech-impaired Children, Association for All (AFASIC), 347 Central Markets, Smithfield, London EC1A 9NH (071 226 6487)

Spinal Injuries Association, Yeoman House, 76 St James' Lane, London N10 3DE (071 444 2121)

Thalassaemia Society, UK, 107 Nightingale Lane, London N8 7QY (081 345 2552)

Bibliography

1. The child

Argyle, M. (1975) *Bodily Communication*. Methuen and Co, London

Atkinson, R. L., Atkinson, R. C., Smith, E. E. *et al.* (1990) *Introduction to Psychology*, 10th edn, Harcourt Brace Jovanovitch, New York

Bowlby, J. (1973) *Attachment and Loss Vol. ii, Separation: Anxiety and Danger*, International Psychoanalytical Library No 95. The Hogarth Press. (Penguin, 1975)

Buckler, J. M. H. (1979) *A Reference Manual of Growth and Development*, Blackwell Scientific Publications, Oxford

Davies, B. M. (1979) *Community Health, Preventive Medicine and Social Services*, 4th edn, Bailliere Tindall, London

Erikson, E. H. (1963) Childhood and society (2nd ed) Norton, New York

Freud, S. (1922) *Introductory Lectures in Psychoanalysis* (authorized English translation) George Allen and Unwin, London

Gesell, A. (1938) *Psychology of Early Growth*, MacMillan, New York

Gesell, A. (with Armatruda, C. S.) (1947) *Development Diagnosis*, Hoeber, New York and London

Illingworth, R. S. (1983) *The Normal Child*, 8th edn, Churchill Livingstone, Edinburgh and London

Inslay, J. (ed.) (1986) *A Paediatric Vade-Mecum*, 11th edn, Lloyd-Luke (Medical Books), London

Lader, M. and Marks, I. (1971) *Clinical Anxiety*, Heinemann, London

Levitt, E. E. (1971) *The Psychology of Anxiety*, Paladin, London

Marks, I. M. (1969) *Fears and Phobias*, Heinemann, London

Piaget, J. (1932) *The Moral Judgements of Children*. Kegan Paul, London

Sheridan, Mary D. (1975) reprinted 1988. *From Birth to Five Years*, Children's Developmental Progress, HMSO and NFER-Nelson. 2 Oxford Road East, Windsor, Berks SL4 1DF

Spielberger, C. D. (ed.) (1966) *Anxiety and Behaviour*, Academic Press, New York

Tanner, J. M. and Whitehouse, R. H. (1983) *Growth and Development Record Charts*, Castlemead Publications, Ware, Herts

Winer, G. A. (1982) Review and analysis of children's fearful behaviour in dental settings. *Childhood Developments*, **53**, 1111–1133

2. *Behaviour management in the dental surgery*

Argyle, M. (1975) *Bodily Communication*, Methuen, London

Barenie, J. T. and Ropa, L. W. (1977) The use of behaviour modification techniques to successfully manage the child dental patient. *Journal of the American Dental Association*, **94**, 329

Elsbach, H. G. (1963) Crying as a diagnostic tool. *Journal of Dentistry for Children*, **30**, 13

Gale, E. N. and Ayer, W. A. (1969) Treatment of dental phobias. *Journal of the American Dental Association*, **73**, 1304

Kent, G. (1984) *The Psychology of Dental Care*, Wright, Bristol

Wright, G., Starkey, P. E. and Gardner, D. E. (1987) *Child Management in Dentistry*, Wright, Bristol

3. *Diagnosis and treatment planning*

Mason, Rita A. (1988) *Guide to Dental Radiography*, 3rd edn, Wright, Bristol

4. *Preventive dentistry*

British Paedodontic Society (1987) Document for Fissure Sealants which included a section on the Clinical Guidelines for the Application of Fissure Sealants. *British Dental Journal*, **163**, 42

British Paedodontic Society (1990) The dental needs of children. *British Dental Journal*, **168**, 79

Donnan, M. F. and Ball, I. A. (1988) A double blind clinical trial to determine the importance of pumice prophylaxis in fissure sealant retention. *British Dental Journal*, **165**, 283

Dunning, J. M. (1986) *Principles of Dental Public Health*, 4th edn, Harvard University Press, Cambridge, Massachusetts and London

Health Education Authority (1987) *The Scientific Basis of Dental Health Education*, A Policy Document, Health Education Authority, London

Jacob, M. C. and Plamping, D. (1989) *The Practice of Primary Dental Care*, Butterworth, London and Boston

Lecompte, E. J. (1987) Clinical application of topical fluoride products—risks, benefits, recommendations. *Journal of Dental Research,* **66,** 1066

Murray, J. J. (1983) *The Prevention of Dental Disease,* Oxford University Press, Oxford

Murray, J. J. and Rugg-Gunn, A. J. (1982) *Fluorides in Caries Prevention,* 2nd edn, Wright, Bristol

Smith B. G. N., Wright, P. S. and Brown, D. (1986) *The Clinical Handling of Dental Materials,* Wright, Bristol

Todd, J. E. and Dodd, T. (1985) *Children's Dental Health in the United Kingdom,* 1983, HMSO, London

WHO (1978) *Epidemiology, Etiology and Prevention of Periodontal Diseases,* Technical Report Series 621, World Health Organisation, Geneva

WHO (1984) *Prevention Methods and Programmes for Oral Diseases,* Technical Report Series 713, World Health Organisation, Geneva

WHO (1987) *Oral Health Surveys,* 3rd edn, World Health Organisation, Geneva

Worthington, H. V., Mitropoulos, C. M. and Campbell-Wilson, M. M. A. (1988) Selection of children for fissure sealing. *Community Dental Health* **5,** 251–254

5. *Control of pain and anxiety*

Davidson, L. and Craig, S. (1987) The use of the periodontal ligament injection in children. *Journal of Dentistry,* **15,** 204

Langa, H. (1976) *Relative Analgesia in Dental Practice,* 2nd edn, W. B. Saunders, Philadelphia and London

Poswillo Report: General anaesthesia, sedation and resuscitation in Dentistry: report of expert working party (1990). Dept. of Health

Roberts, D. H. and Sowray, J. H. (1987) *Local Analgesia in Dentistry,* 3rd edn, Wright, Bristol

Roberts, G. J. (1990) Inhalation sedation (relative analgesia) with oxygen/nitrous oxide gas mixtures: 1. Principles. *Dental Update,* **17,** 139

Ryder, W. and Wright, P. A. (1988) Dental sedation. A review. *British Dental Journal,* **165,** 207

6. *Restorative dentistry*

Clyde, J. S. and Gilmour, A. (1988) Porcelain veneers: a preliminary review. *British Dental Journal,* **164,** 9

Curzon, M. E. J. and Barenie, J. T. (1973) A simplified rubber dam technique for children's dentistry. *British Dental Journal,* **135,** 532

Fisher, N. L. (1985) Restoration of anterior teeth: A transitional approach for the young adult. *British Dental Journal*, **158**, 445

Kennedy, D. B. (1986) *Paediatric Operative Dentistry*, 3rd edn, Wright, Bristol

King, N. M., Bedi, R. and Brook, A. H. (1984) Paedodontics: 1. Isolation techniques. *Dental Update*, March, 91

Murray, J. J. and Bennett, T. G. (1985) *A Colour Atlas of Acid Etch Technique*, Wolfe, London

Plant, C. G. and Thomas, G. D. (1987) Porcelain facings: a simple clinical and laboratory method. *British Dental Journal*, **163**, 231

Simonsen, R. J. (1985) Conservation of tooth structure in restorative dentistry. *Quintessence International*, **16**, 15

Endodontics

Cvek, M. A. (1978) A clinical report on partial pulpotomy and capping with calcium hydroxide in permanent incisors with complicated crown fracture. *Journal of Endodontics*, **4**, 232

Goodman, J. (1985) Endodontic treatment for children. *British Dental Journal*, **158**, 363

Hobson, P. (1970) Pulp treatment of deciduous teeth. Part 1— Factors affecting diagnosis and treatment. *British Dental Journal*, **128**, 232

Hobson, P. (1970) Pulp treatment of deciduous teeth. Part 2— Clinical investigation. *British Dental Journal*, **128**, 275

King, N. M., Brook, A. H. and Page, J. (1984) Endodontic therapy for primary teeth I. Diagnosis and treatment, and II. Materials. *Dental Update*, **11**, 3 (April), 154 and 4 (May), 220

Rifkin, A. (1980) A simple, effective, safe technique for root canal treatment of abscessed primary teeth. *Journal of Dentistry for Children*, **47**, 435

Rule, D. C. (1990) Endodontics for children. In *Endodontics in Clinical Practice* (ed. F. J. Harty), Wright: Butterworth Scientific, Guildford, Chapter 6

Spangberg, L., Engstrom, B. and Langerland, K. (1973) Biological effects of dental materials: 3. Toxicity and antimicrobial effect of endodontic antiseptics *in vitro*. *Oral Surgery, Oral Medicine, Oral Pathology*, **36**, 856

7. *Minor oral surgery*

Howe, G. L. (1985) *Minor Oral Surgery*, 3rd edn, Wright, Bristol

8.   Shared orthodontic/paedodontic problems

Hickson, E. H. and Oldfather, R. E. (1958) Estimation of the sizes of unerupted cuspid and bicuspid teeth. *Angle Orthodontist,* **28**, 236

Houston, W. J. B. (1983) *Walther's Orthodontic Notes,* 4th edn, Wright, Bristol

Nance, H. N. (1947) The limitations of orthodontic treatment: 1. Mixed dentition diagnosis and treatment. *American Journal of Orthodontics and Oral Surgery,* **33**, 177

Tanaka, M. M. and Johnson, L. E. (1974) The prediction of the size of unerupted canines and premolars in a contemporary orthodontic population. *Journal of the American Dental Association,* **88**, 798

9.   Traumatic injuries to the teeth

Andreasen, J. O. (1981) *Traumatic Injuries of the Teeth,* 2nd edn, Munksgaard, Copenhagen.

Bennett, D. T. (1963) Traumatised anterior teeth: Assessing the injury and principles of treatment. *British Dental Journal,* **115**, 309

Ellis, R. G. and Davey, K. W. (1970) The classification and treatment of injuries to the teeth of children. (5th ed) Chicago, Year Book Publishers

Hargreaves, J. A., Craig, J. W. and Needleman, H. L. (1981) *Management of Traumatised Anterior Teeth in Children,* 2nd edn, Churchill Livingstone, Edinburgh and London

O'Donnell, D. and Wei, S. H. Y. (1988) Management of dental trauma in children. In Wei, S. H. Y. (1988) *Pediatric Dentistry: Total Patient Care* (ed. S. H. Y. Wei), Lea and Febiger, Philadelphia, Chapter 17

Welbury, R. R. and Murray, J. J. (1990) Prevention of trauma to teeth. *Dental Update,* **17**, 3 (April), 117

10.   Non-accidental injury: child abuse

Macintyre, D. R., Jones, G. M. and Pinckney, R. C. N. (1986) The role of the dental practitioner in the management of non-accidental injury to children. *British Dental Journal,* **161**, 108

11.   Emergencies

British Postgraduate Medical Federation. Emergency in the Dental Surgery. Video (Produced in conjunction with the Department of Health)

British Red Cross Society (1988) *Practical First Aid,* Dorling Kindersley, London

12. Handicapped children

Court, S. D. M. (1976) *Fit for the Future.* Report of the Committee on Child Health, HMSO, London

Hunter, B. (1987) *Dental Care for Handicapped Patients,* Wright, Bristol

Landsdown, R. (1980) *More Than Sympathy,* Tavistock Publications, London and New York

Maguire, A., Murrary, J. J., Craft, A. W. *et al.* (1987) Radiological features of the long-term effects from treatment of malignant disease in children. *British Dental Journal,* **162,** 99

Poole, D. (1981) Dental care for the handicapped. *British Dental Journal,* **151,** 267

WHO (1952) *Joint Expert Committee on the Physically Handicapped Child,* Technical Report Series 58, World Health Organisation, Geneva

13. Some oral and dental diseases of childhood

Grundy, M. and Shaw, L. (1983) Soft tissue lesions in children's dentistry. *Dental Update,* **10,** 329–590

Jenkins, W. M. M., Allan, C. J. and Collins, W. J. N. (1988) *Guide to Periodontics,* 2nd edn, Heinemann Professional Publishing, Oxford

Kidd, Edwina A. M. and Joyston-Bechal, Sally (1987) *Essentials of Dental Caries: The Disease and its Management,* Wright, Bristol

Seward, M. H. (1971) Local disturbances attributed to eruption of the human primary dentition. *British Dental Journal,* **130,** 72

Seward, M. H. (1972) Treatment of teething in infants. *British Dental Journal,* **132,** 33

Waite, I. M. and Strahan, J. D. (1990) *A Colour Atlas of Periodontology,* 2nd edn, Wolfe, London

14. Childhood diseases

Hull, D. and Johnson, D. I. (1987) *Essential Paediatrics,* 2nd edn, Churchill Livingstone, Edinburgh and London

Insley, J. A. (ed.) (1986) *A Paediatric Vade-mecum,* 11th edn, Lloyd-Luke, London

The Merck Manual (1987) 15th edn, Vol. II, Merck, Sharp and Dohme Research Labs, Rahway, NJ

15. *Prescribing for children*

Dental Practitioner's Formulary/British National Formulary (1988–1990 New edition published every two years). British Dental Association, British Medical Association and British Pharmaceutical Society of Great Britain, London

Lindsay, S. J. E. and Yates, J. A. (1985) The effectiveness of oral diazepam in anxious child patients. *British Dental Journal,* **159,** 149

Appendix A   Norms

Aitchison, J. (1940) *Dental Anatomy for Students,* Staples Press, London

Buckler, J. M. H. (1979) *A Reference Manual of Growth and Development,* Blackwell Scientific Publications, Oxford

DHSS Reports on Public Health and Medical Subjects. No 102 (1988) *The Developmental Progress of Infants and Young Children,* 3rd edn, 5th Impression, HMSO, London

Evans, D. M. D. (1989) *Special Tests,* 13th edn, Faber and Faber, London and Boston

Wheeler, R. C. (1958) *A Textbook of Dental Anatomy and Physiology,* W. B. Saunders, Philadelphia and London

Paedodontics

Andlaw, R. J. and Rock, W. P. (1987) *A Manual of Paedodontics,* 2nd edn, Churchill Livingstone, Edinburgh and London

Braham, R. L. and Morris, M. E. (eds.) (1980) *Textbook of Pediatric Dentistry,* Williams and Wilkins, Baltimore and London

Davis, J. M., Law, D. B. and Lewis, T. M. (1981) *An Atlas of Pedodontics,* 2nd edn, Saunders, Philadelphia

Pinkham, J. R. (sen. ed.) (1988) *Pediatric Dentistry: Infancy Through Adolescence,* W. B. Saunders, Philadelphia and London

Rapp, R. and Winter, G. B. (1979) *A Colour Atlas of Clinical Conditions in Paedodontics,* Wolfe, London

Rock, W. P., Grundy, Margaret C. and Shaw, Linda (1988) *Diagnostic Picture Tests in Paediatric Dentistry,* Wolfe Medical Publications, London

Wei, S. H. Y. (1988) *Pediatric Dentistry: Total Patient Care,* Lea and Febiger, Philadelphia

Index